D1393485

Time to Care

A method of calculating nursing workload
based on individualised patient care

NANCY KATHLEEN GRANT
Ph.D. (Edin.), B.Sc.N., R.N.

The Rcn is very happy indeed to co-operate with the Department of Health and Social Security in publishing this series of research reports. The projects were chosen by the individual research worker and the findings are those of the researcher and relate to the particular subject in the situation in which it was studied. The Rcn, in accordance with its policy of promoting research awareness among members of the profession, commends this series for study but views expressed do not necessarily reflect Rcn policy.

British Library Cataloguing in Publication Data

Grant, Nancy Kathleen
Time to care.
1. Nursing service administration—Great Britain—Case studies 2. Nurses—Great Britain—Supply and demand—Case studies
I. Title II. Royal College of Nursing
610.73′069   RT89

ISBN 0–902606–58–1

Published by
The Royal College of Nursing
of the United Kingdom,
Henrietta Place, Cavendish Square, London W1M 0AB

PRINTED BY THE WHITEFRIARS PRESS LTD.,
LONDON AND TONBRIDGE

Contents

5

7

List of Tables

9

List of Figures

Preface

The calculation of nursing workload is an essential step in determining staffing needs. It would be difficult to find nurses in administrative positions anywhere in the world who are not groping for some method of identifying "appropriate" staffing problems. What is considered "appropriate" depends on one's criteria which are, in turn, related to one's ideas about the aims of nursing. Dr Grant is one of many nurses who feel that the aim of nursing should be the provision of individualised care for patients. Her commitment to this ideal is demonstrated in the book which is an abridged report of her research. It was a stimulating and pleasurable experience to be associated with the work and to observe the growth and fruition of an idea.

A great deal of research has "helpful" by-products, and Dr Grant's study is a good example. Because her method of calculating workload, based on individualised care, required the use of nursing care plans, these were introduced by her and readily accepted by ward staff in several Edinburgh hospitals. The research has been completed, Nancy Grant, a Canadian, has returned to her native Continent—the nursing care plans are still in use.

The book complements several other helpful research reports on the topic of staffing patterns. It presents a novel approach to the complex problem and deserves to be read by all who are involved in the task of determining staffing levels to meet the needs of patients.

LISBETH HOCKEY
Nursing Research Unit
Department of Nursing Studies
University of Edinburgh

Acknowledgements

I would like to thank the nursing staff of the hospital where this research was carried out without whose help this study would have been impossible and who permitted me to observe and time their activities and graciously accepted my presence on their wards.

My especial thanks go to Miss E. Edwards, District Nursing Officer, North Lothian District, who helped me to pave the way for the study.

I find it difficult to express adequately the thanks I owe to my supervisor, Miss L. Hockey. My thanks are also extended to my other supervisor, Dr. R. Daniel.

Finally I should like to acknowledge the financial assistance from the Royal Victoria Hospital, Montreal and the Alumnae Association of the Royal Victoria Hospital.

SECTION I

Introduction

Purpose of the study:

The main purpose of the study is to show a method of calculating the daily nursing workload based on the concept of individualised patient care.

Reason for the study:

As nursing supervisor* in a large Canadian teaching hospital I became aware of the lack of objective information which could demonstrate the need for a certain number of nursing staff. The number of permanent nursing positions appeared to be determined by precedent and by nursing decisions based upon the experience of nursing administrators. Although it might be decided that more nurses were needed, the necessary budget allocation to implement the decision was not always granted. In situations where the nursing establishment could not be met, no information to support any decisions about the possible workloads of staff was available. Thus although it might be considered by the nursing administrators that the workload of the nursing staff was inappropriate for the available nursing staff, no method except unquantified nursing judgment was available for use in discussions about changing the workload.

On a daily basis the number of nursing staff required on a ward can fluctuate due to the physical and/or emotional conditions of the patients, the number of patients and the number of tests and treatments to be performed. No information was available about these daily fluctuations. Although there was a supply of casual duty nurses† who could supplement the permanent nursing staff on a daily basis, these nurses were also allocated on the basis of nursing judgment. Therefore there appeared to be a need for daily, objective information about the nursing workload on each ward in the hospital which could be summed to give weekly and even yearly data.

Nursing establishments in Britain are based on past experience, a fact which is reflected in The Report of the Committee on Nursing:

> No reliable methods of measuring staff requirements have been developed ... there are no generally applicable scientific criteria which can usefully be adopted by nursing and midwifery managers. They have little alternative, therefore, but to bargain, often crudely, for a reasonable share

---

*Comparable with a nursing officer in Britain.

†Nurses working a full $7\frac{1}{4}$ hour day but fewer than 4 days a week. They report to the nursing office each day and are assigned to a ward for the day.

of the budget and to spend their allocation in accordance with subjective judgments related to the circumstances and availability of staff at the time. Since nurses and midwives constitute the largest group of staff in the National Health Service and because they have a major co-ordinating role in the provision of patient care around the clock, it is they who suffer the most from a lack of comprehensive staffing policies within the service.[1]

The need for staffing information in Britain is indicated by the number of studies which have been undertaken.[2,3,4,5,6,7,8] Information about the required nurse staffing could be used:

1. To help make efficient use of the available staff.
2. To measure any difference between estimated staffing requirements and available staffing.
3. To measure changes in the staffing requirements over time.
4. As a variable to be considered in discussions about the quality of nursing care.
5. To provide information both to the nursing profession and the general public.

To expand:

1. Staff could be deployed on the basis of the measured requirements rather than on the basis of professional judgment. This method of deployment would be arranged by nursing officers on a daily basis, adjusting the available staff among wards, taking into consideration the recorded requirements, and by districts and area nursing officers in the deployment of staff between hospitals and the community. The need for this information is expressed in the Report of the Committee on Nursing:

> Within the hospital services the area with the highest staffing level is about 40% better off than that with the lowest; in the community the difference is almost 30%.

2. Measuring any difference between staffing requirements and available staffing can help to influence decisions which affect the required/available staffing ratio. Attempts to adjust this ratio could have considerable effects on other health service departments due to the transfer of activities or curtailment of nursing services affecting the administration of or requirements for other services. If hospital beds are closed due to insufficient nursing staff every other department within the hospital is affected in some way, community services may also be affected if there is a back-log of patients awaiting admission or if patients are kept in hospital for shorter periods in an attempt to diminish the queue.

3. Changes in the workload over time may be due to alterations in administration or practice, which might have implications in long-term predictions about nursing establishments.

4. The required/available nurse staffing ratio should be considered when measuring care given or omitted. If care is omitted it could be

due to lack of staff, if care is omitted when there is sufficient staff, the situation may need further investigation.

5. There is a generally held belief that there is a shortage of nurses.[10,11,12,13,14] The Report of the Committee on Nursing states:

> In studying the evidence we collected about shortages, we were forced to the conclusion that it is not possible to measure shortages without first establishing needs. When shortages are perceived, the underlying worry often seems to centre on quantity rather than on quality.[15]

Many studies have already been undertaken into various methods of calculating nursing establishments; the most recent of these group patients into a number of categories depending on the physical dependency of the patient. By using the average times required for the care given in each category as the basis for calculating the staff required, these methods perpetuate the present practice. The principle underlying the method adopted in this study is unlike the others in that it is based on the workload generated not only by individual patients but also by patients as individuals rather than by categories of patients. It rests on the conviction that patients have individual needs and that the nursing care should be specifically planned to meet these. The workload generated from these individual needs therefore should be measured from the basis of the individual needs. This study describes a system of calculating the nursing workload from such a basis.

CHAPTER 1

Discussion and Survey of Literature Related to the Calculation of Nursing Workloads and/or Nursing Establishments

A workload is the number of manhours required to complete an activity or set of activities at a certain standard including necessary allowances for rest breaks etc. In industry some workloads are composed of time allowances for specific work cycles. However, as nursing is not a series of repetitious tasks, the workload cannot be calculated in the same way as in industry. There appear to be four main differences between industry and nursing which are:

First: Nursing is caring for *people,* and therefore, even if it is subdivided into tasks, nursing workload cannot be confined to a specific time allowance. The components making up each task may be different for each patient due to his individual requirements.

Second: The nursing workload changes daily due to the variety of care required by patients.

Third: Some nursing activities cannot be planned but are determined by nurses' decisions.

Fourth: Events such as emergencies requiring instant attention occur daily.

The activities carried out by nurses and therefore the activities from which the nursing workload arises, can be described as:

1. Those activities involved with assisting a patient with the activities of daily living. Included in this section are basic care, social activities and emotional support.

2. Those activities related to the prevention, diagnosis, treatment and management of disease, such as technical care and patient education.

3. Administrative activities including communication with other departments.

4. Professional activities such as giving or attending lectures and participation in nursing research.

5. Union activities.

The work done by nursing staff will be affected by:

A. The number and type of auxiliary and other professional staff.

The nursing workload is an integral part of the health service workload and is affected by the services provided by other health service employees. There are areas of overlap in the job descriptions among nurses and employees such as doctors and domestic staff.

B. The physical environment, for example: the ward layout.

C. The type of services, such as hospital or community, which may determine the equipment and assistance available. Travel time will be a factor in the workload of nurses in the community.

D. The type of hospital, teaching or non-teaching, with or without a school of nursing, as nurses may have some responsibility for teaching or supervising learners.

E. The regulations of the management which might state activities which may or may not be done by nursing staff.

In short term the nursing workload may be affected by:

1. The number and turnover of patients.

2. The physical and emotional condition of each patient.

3. The number and type of tests, examinations and treatments required by each patient.

4. The demands upon nursing from other departments. These demands could include teaching other health service workers (such as medical students) and preparing patients for and assisting with the examinations of other professional groups.

5. The attendance at educational programmes.

6. The attendance at meetings.

7. Travelling time.

In the long term the nursing workload may be affected by:

8. Changes in standards of nursing care which could be due to changes in method or in the frequency of an activity.

9. Changes in accepted nursing practice due to medical innovations or a change in the role of a nurse.

10. Changes in administrative practice.

11. Changes in the physical environment.

As, judging from the experience of the researcher, any of these factors can change daily, for these factors either short or long term to be reflected in the calculated workload, each nursing activity should be considered daily. This practice could be costly and time consuming but the workload information produced would be comprehensive, consistent and accumulative, allowing for comparisons to be made. The use of the computer for such calculations would seem feasible. Early attempts to calculate nurse staffing were looked at in terms of overall establishment figures. Originally this was done in terms of a ratio of nursing staff to patient beds.[16,17,18] This approach to calculating nursing establishments did not appear to be based on objective information or to take any of the factors which affect the nursing workload into consideration. An important criticism of this approach was expressed by Goddard:

It does not take into account the varying needs of the patient, it includes in its numbers administrative and tutorial nursing staff and indeed it is purely an arbitrary assessment unsupported by factual evidence.[19]

Subsequently, methods were developed which attempted to measure nursing workload on the basis of various factors which affect it. Some methods were used to provide information about establishments, others to measure nursing workload on a daily basis, and some for both purposes. The following review of attempts in Britain to design a method of calculating nursing establishments is ordered chronologically rather than by purpose.

The finding that the difference in the amount of time spent in the basic care of patients is due to the physical dependence of the patient upon which many of the present day methods of calculating nursing establishments are based, was reported in "The Work of Nurses in Hospital Wards" which also stated:

The degree of physical dependence of the patient in any ward has no connection with the amount of technical nursing they may require.[20]

This was a report of a job analysis undertaken to answer the question "What is the proper task of the nurse?" Continuous observation was carried out for one week each on 26 wards in 12 General Hospitals. Work was divided into the following categories:

a) Nursing—basic
    —technical
b) Organisational—contact with other departments
    —internal ward organisation
c) Domestic.

Some conclusions reached in this study were:

1. Nursing should be done by trained nurses not merely supervised by them.
2. Although the medical care of the patient today calls for a skilled technical service from the nurse, it is in the satisfaction of the patient's human needs that her special province lies.
3. Each trained nurse should be responsible for the total nursing care to a specified group of patients—a nursing unit.[21]

It is worthy of note that in 1953 it was considered that nurses should be giving total care to individual patients. The above report did not discuss nursing establishments but the patient-dependency methods of calculating these are based on the finding that the amount of basic nursing care required by a patient was related to his physical dependency.

One of the studies generated from that described above was: "Work Measurement as a Basis for Calculating Nursing Establishments"[22] (The Leeds Study). This study was initiated in order to "study the day to day work of the wards and departments in two hospitals, with a view to determining the number of grades of staff required to satisfy the needs of the patients".[23]

The method used in this study was:
1. Minute by minute observations of the work done in the wards and departments throughout both hospitals.
2. Compilation of a complete job analysis:
a) the work done by each grade of worker,
b) the amount of time spent in each functional area of work,
c) analysis of this time into minutes per bed per work day.
3. Recording the work done for individual patients, classified by the ward sisters according to physical dependency of the patients.

One of the conclusions reached was "that a unit of nursing time, . . ., can be used as an aid to calculating the number of nurses and auxiliary nursing staff required to satisfy the day-time nursing needs of patients in the wards".[24]

The time unit suggested was 125 minutes per bed per day, including 110 minutes for nursing, 10 minutes for personal time and relaxation and 5 minutes for domestic time. This finding was supported by further research.

Another conclusion was: "there is a distinct relationship between the amount of basic and technical nursing done in the wards of like nature",[24] a statement which differs from that made in "Work of Nurses in Hospital Wards"[20] about the amount of technical nursing.

The Leeds study was undertaken to calculate the over-all nurse staffing required in a hospital. The staff allocation to a particular ward would be done on the basis of the requirements of the specialty. The calculations provided information about day staff only, while it is suggested that two nurses per ward are sufficient for night duty.

Calculating nurse staffing from an Index represented progress over the nurse/bed ratio approach in that it was generated from the actual workload undertaken by nurses. This Index did not allow for changes in the dependency rate as this was fixed. As standards of care were not described in this study, the subsequent calculation of an establishment could be based on inappropriate practice which could be due to lack of sufficient staff to implement desired standards or to lack of knowledge of appropriate standards. The establishment figures were based on a single measurement of workload over a set period of time, therefore, changes in any of the long-term factors which affect the workload would make the establishment figures inaccurate.

Wolfe and Young described a method of calculating nursing workload. They attempted to answer two questions:
1. "Given a patient with varying degrees of care needs, how much direct bedside care is provided under current nursing practice?"
2. "How much time is required for all personnel to perform the various tasks on a nursing unit?"[25]

By direct observations it was found that the times required for direct patient care were: self care .50 hours, partial care or intermediate care

21

1.00 hours, intensive care or total care 2.50 hours. In order to obtain an index, the number of patients in each category was multiplied by the time quoted.

By random sampling it was found that the amount of time spent in all other activities for an eight hour shift was twenty hours regardless of the number of patients. The nursing workload, therefore, equals the Index plus twenty hours. Pool staff, that is staff assigned daily from the nursing office, were to be used to balance staff with staffing requirements.

The refinement in this method is achieved by incorporating three categories of direct patient care rather than by using an average patient dependency. Changes in technical care will be reflected in the calculated workload if the amount of technical care required by patients keeps the same relationship to the physical dependency as existed at the time of measurements. Changes in other short-term factors will not be reflected as they are included in the fixed twenty hours. It is particularly inappropriate that such factors as attending classes should be included in a daily average time as classes are not a daily feature. When classes are held, a considerable amount of time may be required for several staff members to attend compulsory sessions such as fire prevention demonstrations. Changes in any factors which affect workload in the long term would not be reflected by using this method, and any such change would render the workload information inaccurate.

Barr[26] described another method of calculating a nursing workload. His approach took into consideration the physical, technical and mental dependency of the patients. Using activity sampling and continuous patient observations, it was found that the ratio of time spent in basic and technical care in each of five care groups was the same as the number of the group. The five groups were:

Care group 1—Self care   with a workload index of 1.
Care group 2—Intermediate care   with a workload index of 2.
               ambulatory
Care group 3—Intermediate care   with a workload index of 3.
               others
Care group 4—Intermediate care   with a workload index of 4.
               bedfast
Care group 5—Intensive care   with a workload index of 5.

Thus group 5 required five times as much care as group one. The information was collected under several headings which included items that might be considered as basic and technical care; in addition there was one heading "Mental State" and another "Extra staff required". The patients were divided into the five care groups depending on their inclusion under these headings. The workload index was calculated by multiplying the number of patients in each care group by the ratio of care required in each group. The data obtained by this method were processed daily for current information on workloads or retrospectively for long-term projections on establishment figures.

Taken into account in the short term but rendered less precise by inclusion in set categories were:

the number of patients,
the physical and emotional dependency of the patients,
the number of specific treatments which were listed.

Not taken into account and, therefore, not reflected in the calculated workload were:

administrative activities,
professional and union activities.

As has been stated previously, certain of these activities do not occur daily but when they do occur, such activities as attending classes or assisting in doctors' examinations can greatly increase the workload.

As the calculated workload was based on the average time spent in each care group at the time of the study, no changes in the factors which affect the workload in the long term would be reflected in the subsequent workload information provided. Norwich and Senior,[27] and Mulligan[28] based their work on this approach.

Two further studies based on patient dependency were undertaken in Aberdeen in 1967[29] and 1969[30] (The Aberdeen Formula). The terms of reference for the studies were:

a) "to undertake investigations at specified departments of selected hospitals in the region in order to ascertain the nursing workload.
b) to determine the duties and responsibilities appropriate to various grades of nursing staff.
c) to investigate ways of reducing the nursing staff workload; either by the introduction of new methods, procedures techniques, or by delegation to non-nursing staff."[31]

Nursing workload was divided into four categories:

1. Basic nursing: the amount of time required for basic nursing was calculated for each of five categories and a factor of 1 assigned to the time required for a totally helpless patient. The factors for the other categories were calculated from this, thus:

Bedfast/chairfast/totally helpless	1.
Bedfast/chairfast/partially helpless	.80
Bedfast/chairfast/but not helpless	.75
Semi-ambulant	.35
Totally ambulant	.30

2. Technical care: the time required was calculated as a percentage of theoretical basic nursing time.

3. Ward administration: the time required was measured in hours per week per patient.

4. Domestic work: the time required was measured in hours per week per patient.

From this basic information a formula was developed. However, in order to simplify the formula, the average dependency and the average number of patients were used rather than the actual number of patients in each category.

Consideration was taken of the physical properties of each ward and layout adjustment factors were provided to accommodate for differences.

An advisory group independent of the research team was given a remit to define an acceptable standard of care. The standard recommended was expressed in terms of the number of basic procedures performed in 24 hours.

There is a danger that the purpose of procedures may be disregarded when the frequency of the procedures becomes the objective. The quality of a procedure is inherent in its purpose; therefore it would seem advisable to state standards in terms of the purpose of the activity. For instance, if the purpose of a daily bath is for general hygiene and comfort but daily bathing dries the skin excessively facilitating the development of breakages of the skin surface, then the purpose cannot be said to have been achieved. Adequate hygiene and comfort in such a case may have been obtained with less frequent bathing but sufficient washing of those parts of the body which become most easily soiled and treatment for the dry skin.

The Aberdeen Formula was devised for the calculation of day duty staffing only, it indicates that for night duty "... the calculation of numbers of staff required, must be based rather on consideration of number required to give adequate service".[32] This statement would seem to suggest that staffing on night duty can be based on professional judgment as was done previously with day duty staffing; but objective information about workload would help in decision-making about night duty staff allocation.

Although these studies described an acceptable standard of basic nursing care, the resultant staffing information would be imprecise if the standards and/or nursing practice and/or administrative practice were changed.

Bryant and Heron described a method of twice daily measurement of the workload of each ward. This method involves recording the physical dependency of each patient and a judgment of the technical nursing required in terms of general, skilled and specialty skills.[33] The information was collected on data-captive forms which can be read by computer. The dependency category of the patient is determined by both his physical dependency and his technical nursing requirements which are based on professional judgment rather than on specific items of care. The use of nursing judgment to categorise the technical care without defining it detracts from the objectivity of the information produced. The authors state, however:

> By making this a professional judgment which involves the nurse in thinking of the whole of the patient's needs, we are certain that her assessment will be less seriously influenced by factors such as shortages of staff or imminent admissions.[34]

The use of this system as described by the authors was: "to monitor short-term variations in patient dependency;"[35] and it is suggested that "the calculations of nursing staff establishment figures necessitates a fundamentally different methodology".[36] However, it might be argued that the staffing requirements to accommodate daily fluctuations must be considered in long-term nurse staffing predictions.

In their study, technical care required by patients was not restricted to a pre-set list but was categorised on the basis of nursing judgment according to the level of staff required under the sub-headings: extensive, moderate and minimal. Therefore, in the short and long term, changes in nursing practice related to technical care were broadly reflected in the calculated workloads. Changes in other factors affecting the nursing workload in the long term were not reflected. Other information provided by this approach was the level of staff required.

Rhys Hearn described "A methodology for exploring the relationships between patients' nursing needs and resources necessary to meet those needs".[37] This approach was originally tried in the United States and has since been used in Birmingham. Both experiences were described. It took into account such things as "reassurance of emotionally dependent patients and the rehabilitation of geriatric or disabled patients".[38]

The nurses' work was divided into three categories of care:
Direct care; care which is patient oriented,
Indirect care; care which is group oriented and
Routine care; care which is policy oriented.

The procedure followed was:
1. Identification of all items of care, categorisation of these items into direct, indirect and routine care. Division of direct care into: support of normal body functions; treatments, procedures, and observations; and professional surveillance, patient education and rehabilitation.
2. Identification of the work content of each item.
3. Assessment of the skill levels required for each item as basic, skilled or technical, which will vary for each patient.
4. Recording of dependency factors such as obese, heavy, incontinent, unable to communicate or unco-operative and movement in or out of the ward.[39]

In the operation of the system nurses were asked to predict:

"1. The patient's likely 'degree of self care' over the next 24 hours.

2. The amount of professional surveillance he was likely to require during the next 24 hours.

3. The treatments, procedures, observations, etc., ordered for the patient.

4. Any dependency factors relevant to the patient."[40]

This information was fed into the computer which had "built-in allowances for probable admissions and discharges".[41]

The output produced was: the patients' care groupings, the predicted admissions, the predicted staffing needs for the three periods of duty and a list of high care patients and their locations.

A daily quality control showed that when the actual staffing level was lower than the predicted staffing level, some items of care were omitted. The first of these items related to ward administration and teaching, the second was acceptable standards of safety, and the third hygiene and general tidiness of the ward.

This approach takes into consideration all the direct care required by an individual patient when placing him in one of five basic care groups and one of five technical care groups. The average time required in each care group was then multiplied by the number of patients in it. Thus although the individual patient is considered in that his care is taken into account, he is not considered as an individual in that he is placed into a category and an average time rather than an individual time is allotted in which to undertake his care. Change in nursing practice related to direct patient care would be grossly reflected in the calculated workload as it will affect the care groups into which the patient is placed but the amount of time allotted to a care group will not be affected. Changes in standards and/or nursing practice other than direct care would not be reflected in the calculated workload; thus the occurrence of any such changes would make the workload information inaccurate. Changes in administrative, professional or union activities would not be reflected in the calculated workload.

An application by the Eastern Regional Hospital Board of nursing dependencies based on three of the studies previously mentioned ("Measurement of Nursing Care"[42], "Nursing Workload as a Basis for Staffing"[43] and "Nursing Workload per Patient as a Basis for Staffing"[44]) provided both information about nursing dependencies and that required by research and intelligence groups.[45] A colour coded nursing record for each patient facilitated the placing of the patient into one of three care categories according to his physical dependency, certain items of technical care and his mental state. At the same time as the nurse recorded the care that the patient had received, she predicted the care that the patient would require during the next twelve hours. From this information the ward officer could calculate the workload for each ward. The uses suggested for this information were:

1. To predict workloads by extending the present workload information over the 24 hours.

2. To establish a code of nursing practice in order to calculate which grades of staff were required for the various care groups.

3. To reduce the workload by recognising premature admission or delayed discharge.

4. To achieve equitable distribution of workload by rationalisation of admission procedures based on existing workload patterns.

This approach considers certain needs of individual patients as listed on the report form but it does not consider the patient as an individual in that he is placed into a group and other care activities which he might require such as teaching, are not specifically included in the workload calculations. In the short term, the demands of other departments and the attendance at professional and/or union activities are not included in the workload calculations. In the long term changes in nursing and/or administrative practice or changes in the physical environment would not be reflected in the accumulated workload information.

Auld undertook her study[46] in a maternity hospital. It is based on the care required by a patient with a normal delivery, the additional care required by patients with complications is considered and the average time for each element of care measured. Twelve precise steps were described by which to determine the establishment.

It is suggested that this method could be applied to other hospitals but the complex diagnoses of patients in general hospitals would seem to make it difficult.

This approach differs from the others in that it categorises patients by diagnosis. It takes into consideration the trends in treatments developing over the past five years. As it was obtained from finite measurements, the information cannot show long-term differences in the workload due to changes in any of the long-term factors.

Summary

Calculating long-term nursing establishments on the basis of a single descriptive study implies that the practices and standards in practice at the time of the study will be perpetuated, which is unlikely. Repetitions of particular studies would indicate changes, but in the interim the actual and the measured workload could have diverged.

The use of the average time required for nursing care activities in conjunction with the average number of patients in particular care categories is satisfactory for long-term projections. However, a nursing establishment must eventually be translated into daily staffing patterns, which if based on these averages would not reflect the actual workload on a given day. Therefore, the daily staffing might be unsatisfactory to meet the needs of the patients on that day. It would appear to be more acceptable to calculate the projected establishment from the accumulated daily workload information.

The most recent methods described for calculating daily nurse staffing requirements are based on patient-dependency. The limitations of such an approach are:

1. The method of collecting data is not sensitive enough to show the effect on staffing of the care required by patients as individuals or to show the amount of time spent by nurses in different activity categories. The individuality of patients is not taken into account, because patients are placed into categories. Therefore, the time needed for any care specific to an individual patient is not considered, thus making the resultant information imprecise. The uniqueness of the patient is further concealed by the use of average times related to patient care. The difference between the time required for a specific patient and the average time could be important; it could happen that the time required for a large number of patients deviates in the same direction from the average thereby substantially affecting the number of staff required.

2. The methods are inflexible in that they cannot accommodate changes in long-term factors affecting the workload without further studies. As this approach of calculating daily nurses staffing requirements is based on current practice it cannot reflect changes in such practice, and therefore the effect of trends and/or modifications in practice would not be shown. For this reason the staffing data calculated would become imprecise. Monitoring of the type and frequency of activities at selected intervals could show changes in practice which could then be incorporated into the system but such a practice would be time consuming and the information provided would still be standardised.

It is suggested therefore that nursing establishments should be based on the information provided from the accumulated daily measurement of the nursing workload calculated on the basis of the factors which affect that workload.

If a nursing workload is the number of nursing staff hours required to provide nursing at a certain standard (including allowances for rest breaks etc.) then the first step in attempting to measure the nursing workload is to describe what nursing is, not only from what nurses do, but from the wider basis of what nursing should be. This provides the content for the next chapter.

CHAPTER 2

The Work of the Nurse

Modern nursing is by no means limited to the giving of expert physical care to the sick, important as this is. It is more far reaching, including as it does helping the patient to adjust to unalterable situations such as personal, family and economic conditions, teaching him and others in the home and in the community to care for themselves, guiding him in the prevention of the illness through hygienic living, and helping him to use available community resources to these ends.[47]

Nursing is defined as a process of action, reaction, interaction and transaction whereby nurses assist individuals of any age group to meet their basic human needs in coping with their health status at some particular point in their life cycle.[48]

The unique function of the nurse is to assist the individual sick or well, in the performance of those activities contributing to health, or its recovery (or to peaceful death) that he would perform unaided if he had the necessary strength, will, or knowledge. And to do this in such a way as to help him gain independence as rapidly as possible.[49]

These descriptions of nursing, written over a period of almost forty years, sustain the idea that nursing is more than giving what tends to be called basic and technical care. The last two descriptions include references to "assisting the individual". Henderson's philosophy[50] has been accepted by the International Council of Nurses (I.C.N.). The important elements in it are: "assist", "individual", "activities contributing to health", "to gain independence as rapidly as possible". Henderson lists 14 needs which might be considered as activities contributing to health, which the nurse may assist the individual to perform. These are:

1. To breathe normally.
2. To eat and drink adequately.
3. To eliminate by all avenues of elimination.
4. To move and maintain desirable posture.
5. To sleep and rest.
6. To select suitable clothing, dress and undress.
7. To maintain normal body temperature by adjusting clothing and modifying environment.
8. To keep the body clean and well groomed and protect the skin.
9. To avoid dangers in the environment and avoid injuring others.
10. To communicate with others in expressing emotions, needs, fear, etc.
11. To worship according to his faith.

12. To work at something that provides a sense of accomplishment.
13. To play or participate in various forms of recreation.
14. To learn, discover or satisfy the curiosity that leads to "normal" development and health.[51]

If a need is uncomplicated by disease processes, a nurse may, if consulted, act independently to help meet the need. If, however, the need is affected by disease process then the nurse will usually act in consultation with a doctor.

Although these needs appear to be discrete, factors which affect one need can affect them all, they cannot therefore be considered in isolation. Needs may be affected by physical factors, environmental factors, pathological factors and knowledge.

Individualised Patient Care

Individualised care may be defined as an ideology of management of the care of a person on the basis of his unique needs, the objective being maximum independence from the necessity of such care.

To assist in the practice of individualised care, the following questions may be considered in relation to each need:

Is there a difficulty in meeting the need?

Does the patient have a perception of the difficulty to meet the need?

If not, why is the nurse's perception different? Are the differences due to: awareness of the situation; theoretical knowledge; cultural factors either ethnical or work oriented such as hospital routines; psychological factors related to the patient's physical state (disease), emotional state, level of consciousness and/or level of intelligence due to age or mental ability?

If the perceptions of the patient and nurse agree, further questions may be asked as follows:

Can the patient meet the need unaided?

Can the patient be taught to meet the need?

Is equipment and/or a change in the environment required to help him meet the need?

Is instruction in the use of equipment required?

If the patient is unable to meet the need, can his family and/or friends meet it?

Do they require instruction either in directly meeting the need and/or in the use of equipment?

Can the patient meet the need with some professional help? Who would be most able to provide this assistance? Will the patient or the nurse do the consulting regarding the assistance?

If neither the patient nor his family nor his friends can meet the need and it must therefore be met by a member of the health team, which person or service is best equipped to meet the need?

The responsibility of the nurse in individualised patient care is described below. The nurse should:

1. Attempt to understand the patient's perception of the need and function on the basis of this perception. Mutual understanding may be enhanced by discussing with the patient, local community or hospital practices. The patient will be better able to implement health practices which can be assimilated into his way of life. If the patient is mentally unable to express his own needs then the nurse must plan to meet those needs on the basis of the patient's culture as revealed by family, friends and/or ethnic or religious group.

2. Teach "acceptable" health practices such as hygiene and immunisation to help improve the patient's knowledge so that he can make better informed judgments about his needs.

3. Permit the patient and/or his family and/or his friends to meet the need. If needs are met for the patient which he is capable of meeting himself, he could lose the ability to meet the need, thus becoming dependent and possibly losing self-respect. Although reliance on family and/or friends makes a person less independent the loss may be less than if he were reliant on professional services.

4. Facilitate the furnishing or equipment or a change in environment and instruct the patient and/or his family and/or friends in the use of equipment. Some simple equipment such as walking aids may be at the disposal of the nurse. The supply of other equipment or environmental changes such as ramps for wheelchairs may require the co-operation of personnel in different health or social services. The availability of such equipment or changes in the environment might allow the patient to become more independent.

5. Assist the patient and/or his family to meet the need. Assisting a patient to undertake an activity detracts less from his independence than doing the activity for him although this may take more time. The patient should be encouraged to participate as much as possible in the planning and executing of his own care.

6. Plan with the patient and/or his family and/or his friends the most satisfactory way of meeting those needs which cannot otherwise be met. This may involve: assembling equipment, executing the activity, cleaning the equipment and recording the activity.

7. Refer the patient to another health and/or social worker if he/she has more expertise in a particular area. The contact might be made by the patient or the nurse depending on the ability of the patient and the current system of referrals.

8. Review the situation constantly and change her activities according to the changes in the patient's needs and his ability to meet them.

The above process of decision making should assist and permit the patient to become as independent as possible as rapidly as possible and may be called individualised patient care.

There is much evidence that individualised care is not practised.[52,53,54,55,56,57,58] Bendall,[59] Schmach,[60] and Boylan[61] discuss the need to change from practising routines to caring for the patient as an individual. This is supported by Lelean:

> The ward routine was shown to affect the care; each patient should be treated acording to her needs and not made to fit into the routine of the ward.[62]

The above references would seem to indicate that routines and the care of the patient as an individual are at the opposite ends of a continuum. At one end, strict routines for the provision of nursing care would be followed and the patient would have to conform. At the opposite end of the continuum would be no routines and the nurse would conform to the habits or customs of the patient. This practice would not seem feasible unless the nurse was employed to do private duty in a patient's home. The placement of nursing along this continuum may be determined by several factors, the first of which might be a belief of the nursing staff as to whether patients should be objects or participants in care or treatment. A second factor may be the availability of staff at certain periods of the day which may be affected by the times when staff are willing to work, the provision of transportation and other commitments of the staff. The times at which patients are served their meals may be determined by the hours worked by catering staff. The time at which doctors make rounds of the patients may be affected by the time at which clinics are held or surgical operations performed.

A third factor affecting the placement of nursing along the continuum may be the environment where the nursing takes place. In hospital the patient is away from his usual environment and may therefore be less in control of the situation. The nursing staff in hospital are in a familiar situation and may therefore be able to have more effect on the planning of daily activities. In a patient's home, however, the nurse is the outsider and may have less control on the time when activities may be performed. The optimum time for effective treatment may also affect the "routineness" of the nursing care. For example, some medications are more effective if given before meals and some if given after meals. If there are several patients receiving medications at the same time a "routine" for distributing medications may have developed. At the other end of the continuum the individual patient would administer his own medications; but in hospital especially there are legal and safety factors which may require that medications be stored under lock. The ultimate in individual care in a hospital might consist of a patient receiving care or treatment when he wants it within the limits of the optimum time for treatment, getting up and going to bed when he desires and receiving individually chosen meals when desired. Conditions suitable for the provision of these activities are not necessarily impossible. For example, for a patient to receive care or treatment when he wants it, depends to a large extent on the number of nursing staff available to give the care. A patient in a single room is able to have the lights and radio on at any time without bothering other patients. The provision of a day room for patients, which some hospitals have, also permits this convenience to some extent. A service of meals on demand is not a feature in most hospitals. However, in a hospital where the patients are assigned to wards according to their physical dependency, in a minimum care ward a cafeteria type meal service might be the most efficient. In wards where many patients require assistance with their meals a more routine meal service might be the most efficient. The provision of these facilities where they do not exist would involve increased expenditure for equipment and/or space and/or staffing.

The number and qualifications of the nursing staff might also affect the placement of nursing along a routine-individual care continuum. If only one trained nurse is available on a ward, her work might become a series of tasks to be completed at specific periods during the day and might be done in a routine manner, because certain tasks may only be done by trained nurses. The work which could be done by untrained staff would be assigned to them. This work could be carried out in a more individualistic manner.

Method of Work Organisation

Another factor which may affect nursing care is the method of work organisation. Some of the various methods which are or might be used in the allocating of the nursing workload are:

1. Task allocation.
2. Team nursing.
3. Patient allocation.
4. Primary nursing.

Task Allocation

Task allocation is a system of assigning nursing activities by specific tasks usually on the basis of the qualifications and experience of the staff. It is thought to be an efficient use of staff in that all levels of staff can be assigned to tasks which they are competent to undertake. Staff working less than a full week and staff working less than a full day, can be easily assimilated. The teaching of pupil and/or student nurses under this system of allocation may be thought to be beneficial in that learners can undertake tasks suitable to their level of training. On the other hand the fact that they do not get the opportunity to consider the total care of the patient may cause difficulties in their professional examinations if they are asked to describe the total care of one patient.

33

Task allocation and practising routines are closely related. The daily routine consists of a list of tasks to be completed at certain times during the day. Therefore, the completion of the task may become more important than the purpose of the task, which is the antithesis of individualised care.

Team Nursing

Team nursing is a system of allocating care in which the staff is divided into teams with a registered nurse as leader and other nursing staff as members of the team. Each team is assigned to a particular group of patients. The patient can be cared for as an individual with each level of staff contributing to that care under the supervision of the leader. For this system to be effective the team leader should be a full time staff member on the same shifts for several consecutive days. It can be a drawback to using this system if considerable numbers of the staff work part-time. A team approach can be useful for teaching student and/or pupil nurses in the total care of the patient and in the direction of other staff members. Team nursing can, however, disintegrate into task allocation within the team.

Patient Allocation

Patient allocation is a system of allocating care in which each nurse is assigned to give complete care to one patient or a group of patients. Under this system each patient has a specific nurse whom he knows to be responsible for this care on a particular day. Part-time staff may not assimilate well into this system, if their period of duty differs from that of other staff, in which case the number of patients assigned to full time staff would vary throughout the period of duty which could create friction. The patients would have two people rather than one involved in their care, thus affecting the coherence of that care.

Assigning the complete care of a patient to an untrained member of staff may be unfair to both the patient and the staff member; the patient may not be receiving the level of care that he requires and the staff member may be undertaking activities for which he/she is unqualified. Obversely, untrained staff members may not be assigned the direct care of a patient but may be assigned to assist a qualified nurse. The feasibility of such pairing of staff depends on the ratio of qualified to untrained staff.

Pupil and/or student nurses working in this system can learn to appreciate the total care of the patient and to organize their own work. It may be thought that this system required more nurses, but the experience on one ward suggests that the system can be carried out with the usual number of staff.[63]

Primary Nursing

Primary nursing* is a modification of patient assignment in which one nurse is responsible for the planning and evaluation of the care of certain patients; other nurses are responsible for the giving of that care when the primary nurse is off duty. The patient knows who *his* nurse is. The nurse, too, is in a better position to know "her" patients and thus to help plan their care; a consistency can therefore be provided which might be lacking in other systems of allocation. This system of work allocation can be useful in the teaching of pupil and/or student nurses as they help to plan both the short- and long-term care of a specific patient.

Because of the various advantages and drawbacks of each system and in relation to the point along the routine-individual care continuum dictated by the various factors stated previously, the system of work assignment in use in any place will be largely determined by the number and mix of staff. A compromise between the various systems may be found to be the most efficient for the practice of individualised care.

The Effect of Individualised Patient Care

Points in favour of the practice of individualised care might include an improvement in the quality of life of patients and economic efficiency for the community. Discussions about the quality of life may tend to be subjective. However, two factors which might be said to improve it are: the relief of pain and discomfort both physical and mental and the aquisition of maintenance of maximal independence. No studies were found to illustrate the effect of individualised care per se but some have shown results of individualisation of care in specific areas.

Healy showed that those patients who received extensive pre-operative instruction had fewer complications, were more quickly on oral analgesics and had more early discharges than the control group.[64] This may have a beneficial economic effect in relation to the number of hospital beds required.

Hayward showed that pre-operative information given to in-dividuals reduced the incidence of pain and anxiety post-operatively.[65] This result illustrates an improvement in the quality of life.

Dumas showed that those patients who had their pre-operative stress relieved had a lower incidence of post-operative vomiting than control patients.[66]

Elms and Leonard showed that "a patient centred nursing approach during admission" is more apt to alleviate distress than approach emphasising attention to administrative tasks.[67]

*Primary nursing in this context should not be confused with the term primary care which may be defined as: the initial assessment, diagnosis and treatment of an individual.

35

Wolfer and Visintainer demonstrated that an experimental group of children admitted for surgery where the children and their parents received "special psychological preparation and continued supportive care" showed less stress than the control group.[68] These results showed an effect on the quality of life through the relief of pain and/or discomfort.

Thierney's experiment in which she used individualised reinforcers in behaviour modification techniques in the toilet training of mentally subnormal patients also illustrates an improvement in the quality of life. It showed that 14 out of 18 patients in the experimental group displayed a reduction of incontinence.[69] This group also showed an improvement in their general level of functioning in relation to other skills. In addition to this improvement "the amount of linen used due to incontinence decreased"[70] and "the workload of the nursing staff due to management of incontinence decreased".[71] These last two results illustrate a potential small economic saving, as a decrease in the amount of linen used will have implications for the amount of linen required and the use of laundry facilities. A decrease in the workload may release staff for other duties or decrease the number of staff required.

More research into individualised care would be useful in showing the efficient use of manpower in terms of quality of life for patients and economics for the community. Such information would have implications in nurse education and in hospital management.

If the accepted philosophy of nursing is one of individualised patient care and if there are benefits to both the patients and the community in practising this type of care, the question arises why individualised care is not practised. One answer advanced by Holder is:

> When nursing was first established the techniques of nursing, and indeed the techniques of medicine, were few and far between. They were basic, they were pragmatic and the real value of nursing was seen in the support, the understanding, care and comfort of the person as an individual. It really was based on a human being meeting human needs.
>
> That was lost as nursing progressed, as medical science and technology increased, as the demands of nursing became greater, as the pace of work increased so that people became more and more absorbed with the tasks they had to perform rather than the people they had to care for.[72]

Because of a generally held belief that there is a shortage of staff, some nurses may be under the impression that this applies to them and therefore that they can only give routine care, although this is not necessarily true. The practice of allocating work by tasks can become a vicious circle; due to perceived staff shortages, learners may be taught task allocation rather than individualised patient care, on the wards. They may therefore consider that task allocation is the recommended method of work organisation; and/or they may have no opportunity to learn how to administer any form of patient allocation. When these learners are qualified, they could then be unable to practise and/or teach individualised care even when there is sufficient staff; consequently the new learners would be taught task allocation as the method of work assignment which would thus be perpetuated.

The question may be asked, what measures are necessary to effect change from task allocation to some other system which focuses on the patient. It would seem that there are two factors which might contribute to such a change:

The first is an understanding of and a desire to practise a philosophy of individualised patient care. If these have been lost over a period of time, the subject of individualised care could be introduced for discussion at unit and/or ward level meetings by the nursing officers and support could be given to those ward sisters who wish to introduce it. Research reports and articles could be used as the basis for such discussions.

The second factor which might contribute to a change in method of work organisation is an appreciation that there is sufficient staff to practise individualised patient care. If the nursing staff do not think that they have enough staff to discharge the perceived workload, whether or not this is an irrational belief, they cannot be expected to adopt new practices which they think will require more staff. If the nursing staff are confident that they have sufficient staff to undertake the present workload, they might be encouraged to try a different approach. To help give this confidence, a daily objective measurement of workload, stated in terms of the full-time equivalent staff required, could be provided to be compared with the full-time equivalent of staff available.

Summary

It has been argued in this chapter that while many nurses accept a philosophy of individualised patient care, and indeed that the practice of individualised patient care may benefit the patient and the community, despite the possible benefits, individualised care is not generally practised. Possibly one of the reasons for failure to practise individualised care is a belief that to do so requires more staff; daily measurement of workload might help to demonstrate whether or not this is so. Such measurement should be based on the care required by each individual patient. The recorded plan of the care required by an individual patient is a nursing care plan; this is the primary instrument from which to calculate the workload based upon individualised patient care.

CHAPTER 3

Nursing Care Plans

A nursing care plan is described as:

> A current written personalised plan for the individual patient. It indicates the kind of nursing he needs, how it can best be accomplished and the goals which nursing personnel hope to accomplish with the patient.[73]

Nursing care plans were originally developed in the United States of America to assist in communication when, after World War II, many non-professionals came into nursing service and team nursing was introduced.[74] The professional nurse planned the care and recorded it in the form of the nursing care plan. The plan could be carried out by non-professionals. Another reason for the development of nursing care plans was the practice of transferring patients from one area of a hospital to another.[75] Sending a nursing care plan with the patient helped the receiving nurse to know what care the patient had been getting and, therefore, she was better able to continue that care.

Since then nursing care plans have been used for assessing nursing care[76, 77] and indeed they are required by the Joint Commission of Accreditation of Hospitals in the United States.[78] They are also useful for educational purposes,[79] because student nurses can, under supervision, plan and record the care of patients.

It must be pointed out that most of the literature concerning nursing care plans originates from the United States and not from Britain.

In Britain, upon the introduction of the kardex system for recording nursing care, it was suggested that nursing orders should be recorded on a form in addition to that used for recording care and placed immediately above it. This practice was adopted in some wards but the orders tend to be written as a list of tasks to be completed. Another method of recording the care to be given to patients is writing lists of tasks each day, such as a list of all the patients who are to have a certain type of treatment.

The care planned for an individual should assist him to become as independent as possible as rapidly as possible. It is helpful, therefore, if the written plan contains the following information:

the specific needs of the patient,
the prescribed ways of meeting these needs,
the objectives to be reached.

The specific needs of the patient could be analysed in terms of the 14 basic needs described by Henderson and listed in Chapter 2.[80] As anything affecting one need may have an effect on others, no need can be considered in isolation. For example, a patient's ability to walk affects his need for assistance with elimination as a chair or bedfast patient will require the use of a bedpan or commode. However, the prescribed ways of meeting needs should not be simply a list of tasks to be completed. Comment on the patient's ability to meet the need and his personal preferences related to ways of meeting the need should be included. For example, rather than, "Hygiene:—bath daily—requires to be lifted into bath"; a nursing care plan might read: "Hygiene—bath daily—to be arranged for $\frac{1}{2}$ hour after analgesics given. Mr. X prefers luke-warm water which he tests with his arm before being lifted into the bath. He is capable of washing himself, except his back, and prefers to be left alone."

Short and long range objectives should be set which can be reached; for example, a patient who is learning to walk with a walking aid may have distance objectives set on a daily basis with a medium-term objective of becoming independently mobile within the ward and a longer-term objective of becoming sufficiently mobile to move about his own home independently. Objectives should be reconsidered frequently as their suitability may be influenced by the patient's condition. Unreachable objectives cause frustrations for both the patient and the nurse.

Nursing care plans are a useful tool for the practice of individualised patient care. This subject has been discussed in Chapter 2. Nursing care plans, moreover, provide a uniform system of recording care to be given. This uniformity is particularly useful if nursing staff move between units in a hospital or between hospitals in a district. If each unit/hospital has a different system of recording, the possibility of errors or omissions due to lack of knowledge about the pertinent system may be increased.

Nursing care plans also provide concentrated information about each patient which makes it easier for staff to locate and hence make use of the information.

Initiating and modifying nursing care plans can be a learning experience for student and pupil nurses. This exercise would enable a learner to consider the total care of one patient.

In discussing the use of nursing care plans some factors which should be considered are:

the purpose of the plans,
the information which might be recorded,
the location of the plans and
the cost of introduction and use.

Purpose of Nursing Care Plans

The main purposes for the introduction of nursing care plans might be to assist in individualisation of patient care. However, there may be secondary purposes such as maintaining a concise history of the nursing care received by a patient. This history may be useful when transferring the care of a patient to another unit or between community and hospital. A nursing care history may also be useful for teaching purposes. If the nursing care plan is to be historical rather than contemporary, there are implications concerning the amount of recording space necessary. A nursing care plan which contains only contemporary information may be recorded in pencil which can be erased as entries become obsolete, thus requiring less recording space. A nursing care plan containing historical information may require more recording space but will give a more complete picture of the care received by the patient.

Another purpose of nursing care plans may be the recording of care required by patients in order to calculate the workload.

The information to be recorded on the nursing care plan may be influenced by the level of independence of the patients. The less independent a patient is the more comprehensive nursing care he is likely to require and the more information will need to be recorded on his nursing care plan.

For ease of reference to the nursing care plan comprehensive care may be divided into categories such as physical needs, social/emotional needs, needs related to diagnosis and treatment of disease and educational needs. The care of less dependent patients may require fewer or no headings.

For community nurses information about the location of a house and the directions for reaching and entering it may be required. All these factors will influence the design of the form.

As confidential information may be recorded on nursing care plans, the location in which they are kept is important. Other factors which might influence the location of nursing care plans are their accessibility to the nursing staff and the physical structure of a ward. In hospital wards nursing care plans may be kept with the nursing kardex in the ward sister's office which may not always be a readily accessible place,[81,82] and, therefore, consideration may need to be given to locating the kardex in a different place or to separating the nursing kardex and the nursing care plans. A nurse recording in the kardex can more readily refer to the nursing care plan if it is with the kardex. However, if the kardex and nursing care plans are together only one staff member can consult them at a time. Therefore, separation may make access easier.

Nursing staff may be reluctant to walk long distances to use the nursing care plans, therefore, consideration may be given in large wards to having nursing care plans located in several places throughout the ward close to the patients to whom they refer.

Location of nursing care plans at the end of each bed may make access easy for the nursing staff but the confidentiality of the information would have to be considered if such an arrangement were planned.

The cost of the introduction and use of nursing care plans will be determined by the saving made by not using the former system of recording care and the expense created by the cost of printing the forms and the purchase of holders for the plans. The use of nursing time may also be a factor. If the previous system of recording care consisted of using several recording books, then the use of one document may appear to constitute a saving. However, the cost of printing in both instances must also be considered. If the nursing care plans are kept with the nursing kardex, no expense for holders would be incurred; whereas using separate holders would initially be relatively expensive.

The effect on nursing time would also depend on the previous system used. However, recording on the nursing care plan as necessary would appear to take less time than recording care for each patient daily.

Use of Nursing Care Plans

In practice, the procedures for using the nursing care plans might be as follows:

On first contact with the patient the nurse could begin the nursing care plan. This would involve the nurse discussing with the patient the reasons which have brought them into contact as well as any observable disabilities and the care thereby necessitated. Other information such as special diet, medications, etc. can also be elicited. After the patient has been examined by the doctor further orders may be added to the care plan. As the patient's condition changes the nursing care plan will be updated. The person making these changes may be determined by the system of work allocation. The ward sister may prefer to retain the responsibility for making changes on the nursing care plan and this would ensure that correct information is recorded; it means, however, that some information will have to be passed from a nurse to the ward sister before being recorded, thereby causing delays. To allow any nursing staff member to make new notations on the nursing care plans should help to give staff members the feeling that the plan is for their use. The ward sister should monitor the nursing care plans and in this way help her staff to make the correct additions. In team or primary nursing the responsibility for maintaining the nursing care plan is delegated by the ward sister to the team leader or primary care nurse. On discharge of a patient the nursing care plan might be kept with the patient's record or it might be sent to another agency to which the patient has been transferred in order to provide communication of all the details of the patient's previous nursing care.[83]

Few people disagree with the idea of nursing care plans but some see problems in their use. One problem is the difficulty that many nurses appear to have in writing a plan, which results in many nursing care plans being inadequate. It is suggested that nursing administrators must give their support if improvements are to be made in this area.[84,85,86] Another problem is the time required to complete the nursing care plan; which also requires the support of nursing administration.[87,88,89] Palisin believes that "nursing care plans are another communication burden imposed on the practitioner by the theorist".[90] She believes that nursing care plans inhibit individualised care. Some of her criticisms may be justified but they tend to be criticisms of the way that nursing care plans are used rather than criticisms of the concept of nursing care plans; for example, nursing care plans may be completed without consulting the patient or the information recorded on the plans may be incorrect. Nurses may not consult patients about nursing care plans because of a belief that patients are objects for treatment rather than participants in treatment. In such a situation the criticism should not be of the nursing care plans but of the attitude of the nursing staff. This situation can only be amended by discussing the attitude of the nurses and the use of nursing care plans. The use of nursing care plans should not be criticised because the information on them is incorrect. It seems reasonable to assume that nurses would commit to paper care that they believe to be suitable; therefore, if the care described is faulty, the mistake is more easily discovered if it is written. The situation can then be discussed with the nurse responsible, and in this way the nursing care plan can prove to be beneficial.

Introduction of Nursing Care Plans

As nursing care plans were seen by the researcher as the resource which contained basic information about the work of nurses from which to calculate their workload, she initially inquired about their use in this country. Nursing care plans in the form described above were not being used in the group of hospitals where this research project was carried out. Some wards were using plain forms for recording orders; many other wards used a variety of books for recording such information as baths, dressings, weights. An ad hoc committee consisting of the Principal Nursing Officer, a medical ward sister from each of four hospitals in the group and the researcher was set up to discuss nursing care plans. This committee decided to design a nursing care plan and test it. The researcher decided that her role in the committee was to act more as a resource person than as a decision-making participant because she believed that the nursing care plan

42

should be designed by the people who were going to use it. The objectives determined for the nursing care plan were:

1. To develop a more systematic way of thinking about and planning for patient care.
2. To provide a standard to assist student nurses to think logically in regard to patient care.
3. To provide a common pattern to facilitate orientation of student nurses around the group and the moving of all grades of staff between wards.
4. To establish on the basis of the information provided about the nursing care required, a nursing establishment.
5. To provide a tool for measuring the nursing care required by individual patients in order to develop a nursing establishment.[91]

It was decided that the care given be categorised under eight general headings, which were: basic care, mobilisation, technical care, individual care, observations, tests and appointments and future plans. A form was designed and given a trial for one month on each of the four wards. Thereafter some changes were made in the design and headings, and the trial continued. The ward sisters felt that the nursing care plan was beneficial and that it should be tried in a wider area. The committee was, therefore, increased to include sisters from other specialties and the nursing care plans were tested on their wards.

The final headings and the description of the content to be described under each which were determined by the enlarged committee were:

Basic Care and Personal Hygiene: type of bath, bed, mouth care and self care or number of assistants, extent of help, etc.

Diet: type of diet, ability to feed self, etc.

Mobilisation: ways of moving the patient and maintaining desirable posture, walking, sitting, lying and changing from one position to another.

Technical Care: procedures to be performed, dressings, intravenous fluids, oxygen, etc.

Observations: temperatures, pulses, respirations, weight, fluid balance, observation of pupils, etc.

Treatment by Medical Staff and/or Investigations: X-rays, lumbar punctures, eye clinic, etc.

Special Needs: problems with communication and how to overcome them, patient and/or family teaching, etc.

Future Plans: plans for rehabilitation, outpatient appointments, terminal care.

See Appendix 1 for the Nursing Care Plan and directions for its use.

It was generally agreed that the nursing care plans had helped to decrease the workload but two ward sisters held the opposite view. It can be pointed out that on one ward seven work books of various kinds were discarded when the nursing care plans were implemented.

The location of the plans was a point of discussion by the committee. It was decided that each ward should determine whether to keep the nursing care plans with the nursing kardex or separately. It appeared that with only one kardex available on a ward, the kardex and hence the nursing care plans were more difficult to consult; this was less of a problem if there were two or more kardeces—proximity of the nursing care plan and kardex was thought to facilitate comparison.

Some advantages and disadvantages of the nursing care plans discussed by the committee were:

Advantages

1. One of the early advantages mentioned was that the night duty staff and staff coming on duty at irregular times found nursing care plans useful. The night staff felt better informed about the activities of the patients during the day and also obtained information about the long-term plans for the patient. Staff coming on duty at irregular times were able to obtain information about the patients while waiting for report.

2. Many staff members felt that the test and appointments section was useful possibly because the information was now in one easily accessible place.

3. It was felt that the plans were of benefit to the clinical teachers as they were able to have a total picture of what the students should be doing for the patients to whom they were assigned.

4. The nursing care plan was seen as a concise picture of each patient and his needs. Some of the information provided in the nursing care plan had been available in other forms but the plan amalgated this information and eliminated the need for re-writing it daily. The nursing care plan provided a structured document uniform throughout the group of hospitals.

5. An additional method of communication was provided for those particulars about a patient which were not always passed along verbally.

6. The nursing officers found it useful for obtaining information about the care of a patient, especially if asked by visitors before having an opportunity to make rounds.

Disadvantages:

1. Insufficient space under some headings was an early and on-going problem in some areas. Different specialties required different amounts of space under various headings, for example: medical wards required more space under Treatment by Medical Staff and/or Investigations than did surgical wards where more space was required under Technical Care. Different designs for different specialties would resolve this problem but the cost of producing different designs would have to be considered.

2. It was seen that the use of nursing care plans could repress oral communication if allowed to do so. It was considered that this should not happen and that oral reports should still be given.

3. The nursing care plan could be dangerous unless kept completely up to date.

The Senior Nursing Officers were kept informed of the progress of the nursing care plans and eventually accepted the recommendation of the committee to introduce the nursing care plan throughout the Region.* They accepted the recommendation and the plans were introduced in all general wards in the group.

Summary

Nursing care plans provide a description of the care which nurses prescribe for their patients, based on the needs of the patient as an individual and the professional judgment of the nurse. Such plans were designed and introduced in the district where this research project was undertaken. Nursing care plans can be used as a source from which to determine the nursing care elements of the workload based on individualised patient care; this process is demonstrated in the next chapter.

---

*This occurred before re-organisation.

CHAPTER 4

A System of Calculating Nursing Workload Based on Individualised Patient Care

In industry the allowed time for an activity is composed of several factors which are: the normal time for the activity, the rest and personal allowance, the process allowance and the special allowance.[92]

As nursing is concerned with people with varying and individual needs, most of the nursing workload cannot be based on an allowed time for the performance of a specific repetitious activity. Few, if any, nursing activities are equivalent in execution when carried out for any two patients. A nursing activity may be influenced by the physical and/or emotional condition of a patient; therefore, the time allowed to undertake a nursing activity should be considered according to the specific needs of each patient. The time required for each nursing activity could be compared with the normal time calculated for an activity in industry. As the time allowed for nursing activities related to the direct care of a patient will vary with each patient and will, therefore, be determined on an individual patient basis, it does not seem feasible to add allowances for other factors to each unit of time. However, allowances can be included in the over-all calculations.

Some of the factors which influence the time allowances for rest and personal time in industry could also apply to nursing, such as: standing, abnormal position, use of muscular energy, close attention and, on night duty, bad light. It seems reasonable, therefore, to allow some portion of the total time for rest and personal allowances.

A process allowance is an allowance of time given to compensate for enforced idleness.[93]

Enforced idleness in nursing could be caused by three factors: waiting for other services, such as meal trays; waiting for equipment, such as waiting for an available bath and waiting for assistance, such as waiting for a second person to help lift a patient. These factors could be affected by the availability and efficiency of other staff, services and equipment.

Special allowances are divided into three sections: periodic activity allowances and interference allowances, which are concerned with machinery or tools. These allowances would relate to nursing only in a small way as generally nurses' tools are relatively simple and major repairs are undertaken by others. The incidence of the use of machines of more complex nature is relatively small except in certain areas such as intensive care units or haemodialysis units. Minor repairs to complex machinery may be made by nurses but any more serious breakdown would probably require immediate replacement of the equipment. The third section of special allowances is contingency allowances; these are allowances to cover "irregular occurrences which are known to happen but whose incidence it may not be possible or economic to study".[94] Irregular occurrences are frequent in nursing, not only because nursing is dealing with people, but because the physical and emotional states of these people may be unstable. Therefore, it is suggested that a considerable percentage of nursing time is required as a contingency allowance.

Nursing workload might be said to include: A normal time and a contingency allowance including allowances for personal time and enforced idleness.

The concept of individualised patient care has been discussed in an earlier chapter. As the practice based on such a concept appears to have benefits for both the patient and the community, this researcher believes that nurses should participate in and encourage its practice. Therefore, a system designed to measure the nursing workload should be based on an ideology of individualised patient care which is the thinking underlying this research. In the proposed system the workload measurement is generated from the needs of individual patients. Such information may be described on a nursing care plan.

The care listed on the nursing care plan is, however, only part of the work which is undertaken by nursing staff; there are other activities such as reports and rounds which occur; these can be called general ward activities. Some of these activities are done collectively for patients, such as serving meals or recreational therapy. Others are supporting activities such as the giving and receiving of reports about the conditions of the patients. Still others, such as serving on committees and attending inservice education programmes, may be carried out for their long-term effects on patient care. Activities listed on the nursing care plan and general ward activities can be called *planned activities.*

Other activities undertaken by nursing staff may be precipitated by a change in the condition of a patient or may be generated by other staff or visitors. All such activities cannot be pre-planned and may be called *unplanned activities.*

The time required for these unplanned activities may be compared with the contingency allowance.

Planned activities may be defined as nursing actions which are scheduled to occur and, therefore, the occurrence and time required for

47

these activities can be recorded, (with provisos about variability in times and occurrence). Planned activities may consist of:

1. Activities which are directly concerned with an individual patient and are listed on a nursing care plan.

2. Activities which are undertaken at planned times for all or a group of patients.

3. Activities related to patient care which are not patient oriented.

4. Activities related to the previously arranged admission of a patient.

5. Activities related to routine housekeeping.

6. Planned meetings.

7. Planned inservice education.

The Time Required for Planned Activities

Activities which are directly concerned with an individual patient and are listed on his nursing care plan might include such activities as: bathing, changing a dressing, assisting with a lumbar puncture and teaching. As indicated previously, the time required for these activities may be affected by the physical and emotional condition of the patient; therefore, the time required for each activity should be considered in terms of the time required for the specific patient according to the judgment of the nurse. This time can be recorded on the nursing care plan. Changes in a patient's condition would necessitate changes on the nursing care plan and could affect the workload. Some factors which might affect the stability of a patient's condition are:

a) the effect of the disease which may be anticipated but unpredictable in detail, in which circumstances the effect cannot be included as planned care.

b) investigations and/or treatments, including surgery, certain effects of which can be predicted.

c) side effects of investigations and/or treatments which are unpredictable and, therefore, the activities generated cannot be included as planned activities.

Activities which are undertaken by nursing staff at planned times for all of a group of patients could include: serving meals, distributing medications and recreational therapy. The time required for various components of these activities could be dependent on the number of patients and/or the number of staff involved; the more patients, the longer the time required. Certain activities require the same amount of time regardless of the number of patients, in which case the time required could be fixed. Therefore, these later activities should be considered in terms of the time required for the various components of the activity.

The total time required for planned activities can, therefore, be calculated from:

A. The time required for each activity described on the nursing care plan. This time is dependent on the condition of each particular patient and is based on nursing judgment.

B. The time required for general ward activities. This time can be calculated by listing, for a specific ward, the activities in this category and determining whether the components of each are affected by the number of patients and/or staff or are fixed regardless of the number of patients. The fixed times can be recorded; the times which are dependent upon the number of patients and/or staff can be calculated by multiplying the time per patient and/or staff by the number of patients and/or staff at the time of the activity.

The total of these times is the time required for planned activities.

The Time Required for Unplanned Activities

Unplanned activities may be defined as: activities which, although they may be expected to occur, are not within the planning control of nursing staff. Therefore, the occurrence of and the time required for these activities cannot be pre-determined. Such activities might include:

1. Communication initiated by others,
2. Informal communication initiated by nursing staff,
3. Activities generated by an emergency situation,
4. Activities generated by an acute change in a patient's condition,
5. Activities generated by expeditious changes in a patient's treatment or investigation plan,
6. Inactivity due to waiting for other services, equipment or assistance,
7. Activities related to emergency admissions,
8. Activities related to the precipitant discharge of a patient,
9. Activities related to general patient observation other than the specific observations described on the nursing care plan,
10. Activities related to personal time exclusive of official breaks,
11. Activities related to the demands upon nursing staff by other departments which might not have been previously discussed.

The amount of time spent in communication which is initiated by others could include either face-to-face conversations, written communication or telephone conversations. This communication might be initiated by patients, other staff and visitors. A visitor may be defined as anyone not specifically attached to a ward, such as staff from other wards or departments or any person from outside the hospital. The number and severity of illness of the patients may affect the amount of communication initiated by others in that family and friends may be more apt to telephone and/or visit to request information about a seriously ill patient. The number of requests for information may in addition be affected by the number of concerned family and/or friends. The number, severity of illness, ability to communicate and personality of the patients may also affect the amount of communication initiated by them. The number of other staff who attend the patient and communicate with the nursing staff may be affected by the number and severity of illness of the patients and the number of other hospital services which they require. Cultural and language factors may affect the amount of communication initiated by a patient and/or his family and friends. In some closely knit cultures many family members remain at the hospital when one of their relatives is admitted. The effect of communication on the nursing workload might be influenced by the availability of auxiliary personnel such as ward clerks or receptionists who would probably screen telephone calls and visitors and undertake the completion of those resultant activities which would be within their control.

Informal communication initiated by the nursing staff with patients, other staff and visitors could be face-to-face, by telephone or written. The amount of this type of communication could also be affected by the number or severity of illness of the patients. The number of other staff involved might depend on the amount of demand for their services which would not only depend on the requirements of patients but also on requests for supplies, repairs or administrative services. Another type of informal communication initiated by the nursing staff might be informal teaching. The amount of time spent in this activity could be influenced by the number of learners and the interest and availability of the trained staff.

The number of emergency situations related to the severity of illness of the patients might be expected to vary with the type of ward; intensive care areas might be expected to have a higher incidence than long stay wards. Emergency situations might include: cardiac arrest, dyspnoea, haemorrhage, extravasation and accidents. Generally such events will add to the workload. Occasionally staff members and/or visitors may have an accident or become ill and, therefore, may require attention from the nursing staff. These events also add to the workload. Other rare emergency situations of varying degrees of severity may be related to internal disasters, that is, a dire situation arising within the hospital such as a fire or a bomb scare. Such events pre-empt the usual work plans and may be handled by bringing a previously planned emergency protocol into effect.

Acute changes in a patient's condition other than an emergency could be the effect of the disease or of investigations and/or treatment or could be accidental. Examples of such changes could be: pain, vomiting, convulsion and depression. The occurrence of any one of these might be a single episode with no other effect or might effect the current plan for the patient's care as recorded on the nursing care plan. Such events generally add to the workload.

Expeditious change in a patient's treatment and/or investigations might be due to a sudden change in the patient's condition or to increased knowledge of the condition through results of tests and/or examinations or consultation. The number of changes in patients' conditions may be related to the number and severity of illness of the patients. The effect of such changes on the workload would be addition to the workload of any time required to undertake the new activities and deletion from the workload of any time required to undertake activities which have been discontinued. The time of day of such changes would influence the extent of the effect on the workload; for example: if the activity is undertaken once a day and has already been completed, then there would be no effect on the workload.

Inactivity due to waiting for other services, equipment or assistance could be compared to the process allowance given in industry. The amount of time spent in unpredictable idleness might be influenced by the availability and efficiency of other services, the availability of equipment and the availability and efficiency of other nursing staff. The system of work allocation might have an affect on the availability of assistance from other nursing staff. If each staff member has her own assignment, assistance might be less readily available than if the staff work in pairs or teams. The ratio of available staff to required staff could affect the availability of other nursing staff to assist with the care of a patient. The availability of other services may be dependent on economic factors which influence the establishment, illness and absence of staff and the workload of the particular service. The availability of equipment may be dependent on repairs and maintenance of equipment, economic factors and the design of the ward.

Unobtrusive observation of patients may be carried out by a nurse walking down a ward or in the process of some other activity. This type of observation is difficult to identify unless a nurse is seen to stop and observe something specific. The amount of time spent in such observation may be affected by the number of patients and their severity of illness. Such observations add to the workload and may generate other unplanned activities. Other non-specific observation of patients is carried out in a hospital during the night when the majority of the patients are asleep but the nursing staff observe for changes in condition and as a safety precaution. This type of observation may be called General Observation.

Staff in industry are given an allowance of time for personal needs; nursing staff have similar requirements. Some work agreements allow for official breaks which may or may not be included in the working hours. If such breaks are included in the working hours a time allowance should be given. If such breaks are not officially permitted the time thus spent would constitute unavailable time; that is time during which the staff is not available for work. It might be argued that breaks are necessary to help relieve the tension created by nursing

51

seriously ill patients. This need might be influenced by the number of patients, the severity of illness and the amount of care patients require. Nursing may also involve heavy lifting which may depend on the size, mobility and severity of illness of the patients. Long periods of standing and/or walking and concentration are also a part of nursing which may affect the amount of rest allowances required.

Occasionally, sudden demands are made upon the nursing staff by other departments which, because of their nature, are accepted. Such circumstances may be due to poor communications on the part of the other department and should, therefore, be avoidable.

An emergency admission may be defined as any admission which has been arranged on short notice or without notice. The effect of such an admission on the workload will be twofold; the work necessary to admit the patient and the work generated by the care required. All people admitted as emergencies are not necessarily acutely ill, so the amount of work created will be variable. Wards of different specialties may expect different numbers of emergency admissions. The number of emergency admissions may be affected by the number of beds available and by the administrative practices which affect emergency admissions. A specific ward may be scheduled to receive emergencies on a specific day or admissions may be assigned to whatever bed is available within a specialty area, hospital or district. Emergency admissions will add to the workload in varying degrees depending on the condition of the patient admitted and the time of the admission in relation to that day's workload. Rarely, an external disaster, that is a dire event outside the bounds of the hospital may occur which generates the emergency admission of a large number of patients simultaneously. The handling of such events supersedes usual practices and a pre-arranged protocol for disasters may be implemented.

The precipitant discharge of a patient may be generated in four ways; death, transfer of a patient, self discharge or a sudden discharge by a doctor. The number of patients and their degrees of illness may influence the number of the first two kinds of discharge. The effect on the workload would also depend on the amount of care the patient had been scheduled to receive. Sudden discharges may be a result of:

Poor communication on the part of the doctor who may have anticipated but failed to communicate an expected discharge.

Important personal reasons may generate a discharge initiated by a patient; this type of discharge is unavoidable.

Unavailability of equipment and/or services due to unforseen circumstances such as a breakdown may generate the discharge of a patient in hospital for a specific purpose related to the relevant equipment. This type of discharge is also largely unavoidable.

Precipitant discharges may affect the workload in two ways; the time required for "laying out" and/or the time required to complete the discharge are added to the workload. The time included in the workload for the care which is no longer required is released from the workload.

As the number and type of unplanned activities are influenced by many factors, it can be seen that the time required for unplanned activities cannot be calculated.

Workload Calculation

The nursing workload will inevitably be unstable because of the occurrences of unplanned activities which are influenced by many factors and because planned activities may be changed after their incorporation into the workload. The effect on the workload of the cancellation of planned activities will depend to some extent on the time of day when cancellation occurs in relation to the time of day when the workload is calculated. Despite these problems, the workload should be measured. Calculation of the workload throughout the day, particularly for the beginning of each shift might give maximal accuracy. However, such frequent calculation would probably involve "real time" computing. The time of workload information collection might be influenced by the time required to collect the information and to perform the calculations, which in turn might be influenced by the method of collection. If computerised nursing care plans are in use, a computer programme could be written to include the other information necessary and to calculate the workload. If computerised nursing care plans are not used but a computer is available other methods of input of the information contained on the nursing care plans and other information necessary to calculate the workload, could be considered such as mark-sense forms, punch cards and keyboard input. In such circumstances and if no computer is available, the information would require manual processing. The time required to process such information and the personnel available to undertake it might affect the time and number of collections. If ward clerks are available, collecting workload information could be part of their job description. If no ward clerks are available then the responsibility of collecting the information would possibly devolve to the nursing staff. As such collections could not be expected to have a high priority amid the work to be undertaken by the nursing staff, collection times could be arranged to fit in most easily with the workload. Therefore, it is suggested that under these circumstances, these collections be made during the night. If workload information is collected during the night fewer changes will be likely to occur before the beginning of the morning shift. Alterations in planned care which occur after this time, other than alterations due to abrupt changes in the conditions of patients, are likely to occur later in the day after doctors' rounds and when test results have been seen. The difference in workload due to alterations in the planned activities will be the difference between the time required for planned activities which have not yet been implemented and/or which have been cancelled and the time required by the activities which have been added to the day's workload. As there may be some balance between these two factors, the actual effect on the workload may not be great. If the balance between the workload and available staff becomes disproportionate, staff may be re-deployed on a short-term basis by nursing management. It is not anticipated that such re-deployment would be required frequently. The workload should be flexible enough to accommodate for some change in work scheduling. The extent of the flexibility may depend on routines which are fixed by factors outside of nursing influence and on the attitude of nursing staff to nursing routines. As this flexibility exists, some work can be rescheduled to suit the availability of staff and vice versa.

It might be said that:

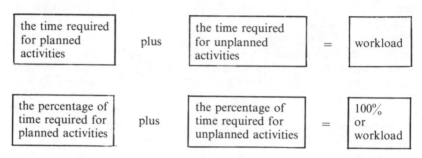

If the time required for planned activities has been recorded and the percentage of time required for planned activities has been calculated:

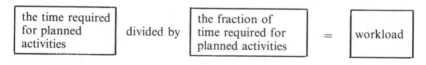

The determination of the time required for planned activities is discussed in Section II, Chapter 6. The determination of the average percentage of time required for Planned and Unplanned Activities is discussed in Section II, Chapter 7. The use of this formula to calculate the workload on one ward is discussed in Section II, Chapter 8.

When the workload is known, the number of full time equivalent staff required to cover the workload can be calculated by dividing the workload by the number of daily working hours of a full time staff member.

There are factors other than workload which could influence the number of staff required, these are:

(a) the necessity of two staff members for certain activities,

(b) the necessity of relief staff for allowed breaks,

(c) the amount of general observation to be done which might depend on the design of the ward, the conditions of the patients and the policies of management.

These factors can be built into a formula for calculating the required full time equivalent staff by taking the higher number of:

the full-time equivalent staff required as indicated by the above three factors or

the full time equivalent staff required as indicated by the workload.

Uses of Workload Information

At ward level, staffing information can be used for planning work on a daily basis. If the full time equivalent staff required is greater than that available, decisions about priorities of work will have to be made. Accumulated data over time may indicate that on a specific ward certain days generally require more or less staff than average. This information could affect the duty rota.

The nursing officer within a unit or hospital upon receipt of the workload and staffing information could re-deploy staff on a daily basis to balance the required staffing levels with the available staff. Pool staff could be used for this purpose.

A long-term discrepancy between the number of full time equivalent staff required and available might indicate a need for discussion about changing the workload or the available staff.

Information accumulated over time about the full time equivalent staff required in a hospital could be used in calculating the nursing establishment. Factors affecting the nursing establishment might include:

1. The number of staff required to undertake the annual workload.
2. Trends developing in the workload.
3. Allowances for statutory holidays, annual leave and illness.
4. Staffing allowances for administrative personnel.
5. Staffing allowances for other departments such as theatres where the workload may be calculated on a different basis.
6. Economic factors.

The ward establishment could be calculated in conjunction with hospital establishment on the basis of the optimum number of staff to give the required staffing cover for a certain percentage of the time. This percentage might be determined by the degree of fluctuation of the workload. The total establishment places in addition to those assigned to a specific ward could be filled with casual duty staff employed as pool staff or to cover for long-term periods of illness and/or annual leave.

The data used to calculate the workload can be manipulated to give other information. The time listed on the nursing care plan can be totalled for each patient to give the amount of time required to give direct care to that patient. This information would be useful to the ward sister for the daily assigning of work among the nursing staff.

The amount and percentage of planned time spent in each work category can be calculated. The amount and percentage of time should be considered together as the percentage may fluctuate due to changes in other categories while the amount of time remains relatively the same. Daily differences would be expected to occur as some activities are not daily occurrences; therefore weekly calculation is suggested. Over time changes and trends in the amount and percentage of planned time in the various categories would be illustrated. On a specific ward, innovations in practice might result in a different proportion of time being spent in some activity; if such changes are due to policy change, the effect on the workload could be demonstrated by these measurements. If unexpected changes are demonstrated, it may be desirable to discover the reasons for them.

Differences in the percentage of time spent in various work categories on different wards could be due to the type of ward; surgical wards might be expected to spend more time in the technical category than medical wards. The priorities set by the ward sister and/or staff would also be reflected in the amount and percentage of time spent in various categories of care. Therefore, two or more similar wards could be compared as to the amount and percentage of time spent in certain categories compared with patient satisfaction, job satisfaction, etc.

Hospital nursing staff may cover two or three shifts, and so the workload should be calculated for each shift. On day duty the workload may be relatively evenly spread over the shift. This is not so on night duty, when there may be more planned work at either or both ends of the shift. The amount of this work may depend on the length of the shift and the structure of the patients' day. During the middle of the night the majority of patients may be expected to be asleep and few activities are planned. At this time the staff undertake general observation, the amount of time for which may be influenced by:

the minimal degree of observation required,

the number of nurses available for additional observation on night duty,

the design of the ward,

the ability of patients to signal to the nursing staff.

Because of the irregular pattern of work on night duty it may be necessary to examine the workload in two sections; first, those parts of the night when the greatest part of the planned work is undertaken and secondly, the middle of the night when it is expected that there are fewer planned activities. Possible ways of managing the irregular pattern of work on night duty might be:

(a) To change the shift pattern by having a shorter night shift. The bulk of the planned work might be undertaken before the night staff come on duty and after they go off duty.

(b) To have an overlap of staff between the day and night shifts during the time in which planned activities occur.

(c) To change the pattern of the patients' day, especially with regard to care given early in the morning. The time when this care is given depends to some extent on the time at which breakfast is served, which in turn determines the time at which patients are awakened.

When calculating staffing hours available it may be important to give special consideration to two types of staff members, ward sisters and learners.

Some of the activities undertaken by the ward sister differ from those of her staff. Such activities might include: arranging duty hours, assessing staff, orienting and teaching staff. It might also be expected that the ward sister would engage in or be engaged in more communication than other nursing staff. Therefore, the ward sister cannot be considered as being available to undertake the workload thus measured, for her full period of duty. She should be permitted some time to undertake her unique duties, indeed, the Leeds study suggested that only 20% of the ward sister's time should be considered available to undertake "actual nursing duties".[95] Some factors which might affect the amount of time which the ward sister requires for her unique duties might be:

Arranging duty hours:

the system used for arranging duty hours which might be a fixed rotation system or the duty hours may be planned weekly or monthly,

the number of staff to be assessed,

the number of staff to be oriented and taught, including learners,

the availability of clinical instructors,

the number of patients and other staff with whom communication is required.

Student and pupil nurses by virtue of their learning roles are not comparable to full time equivalent staff. The amount of time which they require to undertake an activity may be affected by their degree of skill and the fact that they are being instructed. Their degree of skill and/or management policy might also dictate which activities they may undertake. This restriction might not affect the workload if there is an optimum balance of trained staff and learners but if there is an imbalance in this ratio, the workload could be affected. Therefore, it is suggested that rather than being counted as full time staff, a learner should be counted as a percentage of a full time staff member. This percentage would require to be calculated from the additional time required by learners.

Summary

A system of measuring nursing workload based on the philosophy of individualised patient care has been described. The workload is based

57

on the amount of time required for planned activities plus a percentage of time for unplanned activities. From this basic workload other information can be calculated.

CHAPTER 5

Selection of a Hospital Ward and Obtainment of Permission to Undertake the Study

The project was designed to test whether the suggested system could be operationalised. For this purpose the following steps were taken.

1. Selection of a hospital ward and obtainment of permission to undertake the study.
2. Determination of the time required for planned activities.
3. Determination of the percentage of time spent in planned and unplanned activities.
4. Introduction and operation of the system by the researcher.
5. Operation of the system by the ward staff.
6. Extension of the system to other areas.

Selection of Hospital Ward.

There were two major factors to be considered in selecting the hospital, the location of the hospital and the use of a nursing care plan.

As it was important not to "over research" a particular hospital and as other research was known to be in progress in various hospitals, it was important to select a hospital in which this project would not interfere with on-going work.

The location of the hospital was also important for financial and transport reasons. The hospital had to be near public transport, ideally within the city limits.

As the system required the use of nursing care plans for recording of the care required by a patient, it was important that the hospital selected used or was willing to use nursing care plans.

It was preferable that the ward be a medical one as the researcher was more familiar with medical nursing practice.

Permission to Undertake the Study

Permission to initiate the study was easily obtained. A local Principal Nursing Officer was approached by letter for assistance concerning a period of orientation to British nursing for the researcher and for information about nursing care plans. In the ensuing discussion it was decided to set up the committee to discuss nursing care plans described in Chapter 3. The Principal Nursing Officer also supported the request to the Chief Area Nursing Officer to do the research in one of the hospitals in the group; this request was granted.

Having obtained general permission to undertake the research project, one of the ward sisters serving on the Nursing Care Plan Committee was approached by both the Principal Nursing Officer and the researcher for permission to undertake the study on her ward. This request was also granted. The Senior Nursing Officer, having been kept informed of the situation by the Principal Nursing Officer, was apprised of the research in more detail.

The ward selected was a 39 bed acute medical ward in a teaching hospital with both student and pupil nurses. The ward was situated on two floors and consisted of 5 patients' rooms.

The beds were in theory divided in the following way:

23 medical beds—8 male and 15 female,

16 convalescent gynaecological beds.

However, in practice only 8 beds were used for convalescent gynaecological patients and the other 8 gynaecological beds were used for medical patients.

The nurses worked three shifts divided into two periods: day duty and night duty. The hours worked by full time staff were:

07.30–16.30   early day duty

12.00–21.00   late day duty

For the purpose of calculation of required staffing hours the two day duty periods were combined. Two unpaid half-hour meal breaks were allowed on each shift and a 15 minute tea break on the late day shift.

The work assignment was generally by task allocation although the assignments were routine rather than specifically allocated. An exception to this situation was giving baths and making beds in the morning, when two or more nurses were assigned to a room or rooms. Other routine tasks during the day might be generally done by one grade of staff because of training or lack of training. For example, nursing auxiliaries do not take blood pressures and were, therefore, excluded from this task, otherwise all grade of staff assisted each other.

It has been suggested in Chapter 2 that task allocation detracts from individual care. As this study was undertaken to investigate a method of calculating nursing workload based on individualised patient care, it might be thought that a ward practising task allocation would not be a suitable environment in which to undertake this study. However, as individualised patient care is an ideology and not a work prescription, it is the theory of the system of calculating nursing workload which is based on individualised patient care; in practice the method should apply to any type of work prescription. It was not the intention of the researcher to influence either the ideology or the type of work prescription in the place where the study was carried out although it is realised that discussions about nursing care plans and individualised patient care might have some effect on the situation.

The ward staff was told in detail about the research and their individual permission was requested to measure the amount of time that they spent in various activities. This was a continuous process as there was a turnover of both permanent staff and learners. Therefore, as each new staff member came to the ward she was told about the research project and was asked for permission to be observed and to have her activities timed. There were no refusals. In order to preserve anonymity, the staff were coded by number.

Patients had the research project explained to them at the time of the observations. It was impossible to do this in advance due to the turnover of patients. As the focus of observation was the activities of the nursing staff and not the patients, it was not thought necessary to obtain the consent of the patients although they were on the whole informed about the research. Some patients were deemed too ill for this but the majority of patients were told and there were no objections.

CHAPTER 6

Determination of the Time Required for Planned Activities

A variety of possible methods of eliciting the amount of time required for planned activities was considered. These were:

A. Other studies of nursing workload might provide records of the amount of time required for certain activities. As ward design, provision of equipment and usual practices may be expected to vary from hospital to hospital, it was expected that such information might not adequately reflect the amount of time required for activities in the ward studied.

B. The nursing staff practising the activity could be considered as a panel of experts and consulted about the time requirements for activities. This method was discarded for the following reasons: First, it was possible that the nursing staff would think in terms of elapsed time,* not in man hours.** Secondly, in order to use this method, it would have to be established that each respondent was using the same definition for each activity. The third reason for discarding this method was the difficulty of determining adequately the timing per patient when this was relevant.

C. The times required for certain activities might be recorded with the printed descriptions of these activities. It was thought that the School of Nursing might be able to provide this specific information, however, it was found not to be the case.

D. The time taken for activities could be observed and recorded. This method would be more time consuming than any of the other methods considered; however, it would give more precise details about the

---

* Elapsed time is the amount of time from the beginning to the end of an activity excluding interruptions.
** Man hours are the total amount of time expended by all staff involved in an activity.

ward. The times determined in this way would reflect the practices in effect and the physical structure of the ward.

The last method was adopted.

Factors to be Considered in Measuring the Time Required for Planned Activities

Factors to be considered in measuring the time required for planned activities are:

A. The definition of each activity,
B. The area of observation,
C. The factors which could affect the amount of time taken,
D. The number of observations to be made,
E. The equipment to be used by the researcher.

The Definition of each Activity

In order to measure the amount of time taken for an activity it was necessary to have a definition of each activity. For this reason, copies of the available descriptions of nursing procedures were obtained from the School of Nursing. These were not found to be suitable as they did not contain directions for some of the more frequent activities such as giving baths or taking temperatures. For this reason and because it was thought that even within activities there might be differences which could affect the amount of time required, it was decided to describe and time activities and classify them later.

A decision had to be made regarding the beginning and end of each activity which required some appreciation as to the type of activity. There were three factors which assisted in determining what type of activity was about to start. One factor was nursing judgment. The researcher was a qualified nurse with several years nursing experience including four years as chairman of a procedure committee. Other factors were the ward routine and conversations by the ward staff which indicated the activity about to start. An activity was judged to begin and hence timing was commenced, when: (a) a staff member or members approached a patient to begin an activity, (b) a staff member or members started to obtain the equipment necessary, (c) the appropriate staff met for an activity in which no patients were involved.

The completion of an activity might be indicated by the commencement of another activity by the nursing staff involved or by the recording of the activity and/or replacement of the equipment. However, any activity might be discontinued temporarily, for example: when a patient was given a basin for washing, the nurse could distribute other basins while the first patient was washing, then return to remove and clean the first basin. The actual completion of an activity was based on nursing judgment. A bath, for example, was

63

considered to be completed when the patient's bed was made, his unit tidied and the patient returned to a suitable location dressed in day clothes, if appropriate. Attention to hair and nails were included in the activity if they were undertaken. The aggregate of an activity might include talking with the patient, preparing equipment, performance of the activity, cleaning and replacing equipment and recording the activity. Observations which were similar in content were grouped and defined as an activity.

The Area of Observation

Some nursing activities might be undertaken by more than one staff member. In such an event the various staff members concerned might be in different locations, for example, one staff member may have prepared the bath while another assisted the patient to walk to the bath. Therefore, it was necessary to site the observer where she could at least be aware of the location of all staff participants even if she was not able to see them. Bedside curtains are drawn for some activities and other activities occur behind closed doors. If the observer was sited behind the curtains or doors it would have detracted from patient privacy and a person extraneous to the needs of the patient would have been present at interactions taking place between the patient and staff member: this situation might have inhibited discussion. If the observer was behind bedside curtains or doors the amount of space available to the nursing staff in which to undertake the activity would have been decreased. When any staff member left the enclosed area the observer would have had to follow in order to note if that staff member was continuing with the activity or taking up another; this movement into and out of the area might have been distracting for both the patient and the staff. Therefore, it was decided that the observer should not intrude behind the bedside curtains or behind closed doors. This position would detract from observation of the part of the activity occurring behind the curtains but it would permit better observations of the part of the activity occurring outside the curtain.

The Factors which could Affect the Amount of Time Taken

The amount of time required to undertake an activity may be affected by several factors. These are:
  (i) the amount of training and experience of the staff member undertaking the activity,
 (ii) the condition, age and sex of the patient,
(iii) the design of the ward,
 (iv) the equipment available,
  (v) the standard of care,
 (vi) the effect on the staff of being observed.

(i) It was expected that learners would take longer to complete an activity which was new to them or if they were being instructed or supervised for an activity. Therefore, it was decided where possible not to observe learners on their first ward or other learners who were being taught, supervised or doing activity for the first time. It was not possible to omit these learners if they joined an activity already in progress or when the activity was one in which all staff participated such as serving meals.

(ii) The fact that the condition, age and sex of a patient may affect the time required for an activity has already been discussed. As the amount of time determined for activities which would be so affected was for a guideline only, it was acceptable that the measurements be affected by these factors.

(iii) Individual wards might have different designs and therefore, the amount of time required to obtain and/or set up equipment may vary from ward to ward. As only one ward was under observation this factor would be included in the amount of time measured for an activity on that ward.

(iv) Factors such as variable height beds might affect the amount of time required. On a ward where only one type of a piece of equipment was used, the effect of the equipment would be included in the work time measured. Where different types of a piece of equipment existed on one ward it would be desirable to determine separately the amount of time taken using each type of equipment.

(v) The observer was not able to judge the needs of any patients; therefore, she was unable to determine the standard of care given. The definition of a particular activity depended on the number of observations of an item of care which contained the same elements; if an item of care was observed only once or twice to be done in a certain way, it would not be constituted as an activity. If the content of an activity was frequently observed to be similar it would be constituted as an activity. In this way the present standards of care related to the completeness of an activity were incorporated into the definition of the activity.

(vi) Possible reactions to be expected from the staff due to being observed might be:

an increase in the speed at which work is performed due to nervous reaction or to demonstrate "efficiency",
a decrease in the speed at which work is performed due to a negative reaction to "work study",
a decrease in the speed at which work is performed due to a desire to maximise the amount of time allowed for an activity,
a decrease in the speed at which work is performed due to a desire, conscious or unconscious, to improve the "quality of care",
no change in the speed at which the work is performed.

In order to minimise the effect of an increase or decrease in the speed at which work was performed, the first three days of observation were discarded as it was expected that any change in the speed of work would not be continuously maintained. This practice also allowed time for the observer to gain experience.

The Number of Observations to be Made

Two factors which influenced the number of observations of each activity were; first, that only one observer, the researcher, was available. As realistically she could only observe for a limited period in any one day, it was decided that observations would take place at the convenience of the researcher but covering the 24 hours of the day. In this way an activity which occurred once in 24 hours could be observed. The second factor affecting the number of observations made was that some activities would be undertaken more frequently than others. Some activities such as baths tend to be daily events and some activities such as taking temperatures tend to occur more frequently. These types of activities would be easily observed. Other activities such as wound dressings occur less frequently; therefore it would be difficult, if not impossible, to obtain many observations of this type of activity. It was decided initially to observe at least ten incidents of each activity with the exception of those activities which occurred so infrequently as to make this impossible.

The Equipment to be Used by the Researcher

It was decided to measure the time taken for an activity to the nearest minute. It was thought that greater accuracy would be difficult to achieve particularly for activities undertaken simultaneously by two or more staff members. The timings determined to be used as guidelines only, did not appear to require accuracy greater than to the nearest minute. The watch used to measure the time could have been either a stop-watch or an ordinary wrist-watch. As a stop-watch would have added to the costs and as the degree of accuracy provided by using a stop-watch was not required, it was decided to use a wrist-watch. No extra cost was involved and sufficient accuracy could be obtained. A wrist-watch would be easier for the observer to use and it was thought that it would be less threatening to the staff under observation.

The only other equipment needed was a clipboard to support the collection forms.

The Collection of the Data

The information collected in order to determine the time required for planned activities was:

66

the date, to help identify each observation,
the time to the nearest minute at which a staff member commenced, joined, left or finished an activity,
the code number of the staff involved to compare the time required by different staff members and different levels of staff,
the bed number or hospital number of the patient involved, to compare the time required by different patients,
a description of the activity, to aid in defining the activities.

The amount of time required for an activity may be measured in elapsed time or in man hours. The elapsed time was calculated when the activity was not influenced by the number of staff; for example, giving the change of shift report required the same amount of time whether given to three or five staff members. Man hours were calculated when the elapsed time was affected by the number of staff who were undertaking the activity; for example, serving the tea took less elapsed time if undertaken by two staff members than if it were undertaken by one. When either of these measurements was affected by the number of patients; for example, the amount of time required for both giving report and serving tea depended on the number of patients involved. The number of patients was not involved when setting up trolleys for serving meals.

Copies of one period of the information recorded for one day duty period is shown in Appendix 2.

Occasionally the observer missed an observation, in this event, these observations were discarded. The completed observations were transferred to another form in order to calculate the amount of time spent by each participant in each activity and the total time taken for an activity. The information was then transcribed to an individual form for each activity such as the one for Rounds with the night charge nurse shown in Table 1. Ten observations of this activity were made. Although two staff members participated the amount of time was not affected by the number of staff participating. However, the number of patients might have affected the amount of time taken, therefore, the elapsed time was divided by the number of patients. No mode appeared; therefore, the mean of .22 minutes per patient was accepted as the amount of time required for the day and night charge nurses to make rounds of all the patients in the morning.

As was expected, the amount of time measured for some activities varied considerably. Possible reasons for such differences are those listed in this chapter as factors which could affect the amount of time taken.

As in many activities various grades of staff worked together, it was not possible to determine if the amount of training or experience affected the amount of time taken. Other activities were generally undertaken by one grade of staff. Exceptions to this situation were the activities entitled: "Turn patient", "Feed breakfast and supper", and

"Blood pressures". The amounts of time taken for all of these activities by different grades of staff were similar although the number of examples was too small for statistical analysis. Therefore, no conclusions could be drawn about the effect on the amount of time taken for an activity when it is done by different grades of staff.

Statistical Measures Used

For each of these activities the Mean, Mode, Median and Standard Deviation were calculated. When a mode of more than one unit existed it was selected either as the figure for the suggested amount of time provided to assist the nursing staff in making judgments about the amount of time required for a specific patient or as the fixed time per patient/per activity for general ward activities. When no mode or a mode of only one unit existed the mean was used for the same purposes.

Table 2 shows the measurements of the amount of time taken to weigh a patient who was capable of getting on and off the scales without assistance. This example demonstrates an activity done by one staff member; hence, the elapsed time was used for the calculations. As a mode of 2 minutes was demonstrated, the amount of time suggested

TABLE 1

Form used for Recording the Amounts of Time Observed of "Rounds with the Night Charge Nurse" and Subsequent Calculation of the Amount of Time to be Ascribed to this Activity when Calculating the Workload.

Date	Observation number	Staff code	Elapsed time in minutes	Number of patients	Elapsed time in minutes ÷ patients	Any relevant additional information
19 July	1	1, ?	6	28	.21	
6 Aug.	1	1, ?	4	21	.19	
28 Sept.	1	1, ?	8	29	.28	
23 Oct.	1	62, ?	5	27	.19	
2 Nov.	1	1, ?	6	26	.23	
14 Dec.	1	1, ?	6	25	.24	
16 Jan.	7	4, 36	7	38	.18	
18 Jan.	9	3, 42	7	39	.18	
24 Jan.	16	1, 36	9	39	.23	
25 Jan.	15	1, 42	11	35	.31	
Mean					.22	
Mode					—	
Median					.22	
Standard Deviation					.05	

TABLE 2
Amount of Time Taken to Weigh a Patient Capable of Getting on and off the Scales Unaided.

Weight: Bring scales to patient, patient on/off scales without help, record weight, return scales or take to another patient.

Date	Staff code	Patient bed or hospital number	Elapsed time in minutes	Any relevant additional information
1 May	4	$1^{(6)}$*	1	
23 May	27	71011	3	
23 May	27	71267	2	
23 May	27	$2^{(2)}$	4	
1 June	21	7409	2	
8 June	27	71267	2	
8 June	27	14293	2	
8 June	27	71709	1	
12 June	30, 28	7409	2	
29 June	10	$2^{(2)}$	3	
19 July	4	72175	4	
23 Oct.	62	$2^{(4)}$	2	
Mean			2.3	
Mode			2	
Median			2	
Standard Deviation			.97	

*Bed number, i.e. Room 1, Bed 6

for this activity was 2 minutes. The median and mean (if taken to the nearest minute) were identical to the mode.

Table 3 shows the measurements of the amounts of time taken to bath a patient in bed when the patient remains in the bed while the bed is being made.

The amount of time taken for this activity is affected by the number of staff; therefore, man hours were used for the calculations. There was no mode but the mean and median were within one minute if taken to the nearest minute. The guideline for this activity was 33 minutes.

Table 1 shows the measurements of the amount of time taken to make rounds of all the patients by the night and early day charge nurses. The amount of time taken for this activity is affected by the number of patients but not by the number of staff. Although two staff members are involved it must be noted that each is working on a different shift. As this was a General Ward Activity the time was fixed. There was no mode, the mean and median were identical, therefore, the

TABLE 3
Amount of Time Taken to Bath a Patient in Bed when the Patient Remains in Bed.

Bed Bath: Bath a patient in bed, make bed with patient in it.

Date	Staff code	Patient bed or hospital number	Man minutes	Any relevant additional information
10 May	26,8	$2^{(2)}$	26	
15 May	27,9	71433	22	
18 May	6,23	$2^{(2)}$	48	Patient had intravenous infusion
22 May	26,29	$2^{(2)}$	40	Patient had intravenous infusion and oxygen
23 May	27,1 5	$2^{(6)}$	38	Acutely ill, nasogastric tube, suction
5 June	22,25	71684	48	
16 July	1,46	$2^{(1)}$	22	
19 July	1,29	$2^{(7)}$	16	
19 July	6,45	71495	39	
6 Aug.	32,10	72314	29	
Mean			32.8	
Mode			—	
Median			33.5	
Standard deviation			10.75	

amount of time fixed for this activity was .22 minutes per patient on both day and night shifts.

The amounts of time required for 42 activities were determined from at least 10 observations; the amounts of time suggested for 24 other activities were derived from less than ten observations. All results were discussed with the Ward Sister who agreed with all but one. The exception was to be used as a guideline only and the amount of time indicated for the activity was not changed.

The amounts of time required for other activities which had not been observed were discussed with the Ward Sister and suggested amounts of time set, either on the basis of the number of observations made and/or professional judgments. All these activities involved direct care to the patient.

A list of the times determined for activities is shown in Appendix 3.

Summary

Planned Activities were divided into two sub-categories: those activities listed on a Nursing Care Plan and General Ward Activities.

The amount of time required for activities listed on the Nursing Care Plan was to be determined by the nursing staff. However, in order to assist in these decisions, the modal or mean times taken to complete these activities were listed. These times were based on at least ten observations. The amount of time required for General Ward Activities was based on the modal or mean times taken to complete these activities, based on at least ten observations. The times for those activities which were not observed ten times were based on professional judgment.

CHAPTER 7

Determination of the Percentage of Time Spent in Planned and Unplanned Activities

There were two possible ways of measuring the percentage of time spent in Planned and Unplanned Activities: activity sampling and continuous observation. Activity sampling might give more information as more staff members would be included in the observations but due to the many interruptions to nursing activities might be less accurate. Also, it might be difficult for the observer to differentiate between Planned and Unplanned Activities on short observation. Continuous observation would give less information in that fewer staff members would be observed but the information might be more accurate. Therefore, it was decided to use continuous observation.

The amount of time available for observation was limited by the fact that only one observer, the researcher, was available. Because of this restriction and, in order to obtain the broadest picture of the ward possible, it was decided to observe each permanent member of the ward staff for one complete period of duty. The exception to this plan was the Ward Sister; as her job was seen as being unique it was decided to observe her on five occasions. Learners, not on their first ward, who had been on the ward for more than one week which would allow them to become accustomed to the presence of the observer, were also to be observed.

To have observed each staff member for less than a complete period of duty would have provided a less accurate description and would have required more time. An activity could take place at different times on different days. If the period of observation of a staff member was divided over several days, the same daily activity might be observed on more than one occasion. This circumstance would have increased the apparent amount of time in Planned Activities. Therefore, it was decided to observe each staff member over their complete period of duty.

Each member of staff was approached individually for permission to obtain and time her activities. There were no definite refusals although there was one request not to observe a staff nurse when she was in charge of the ward but permission was given to observe her when she was not in charge.

On day duty, 12 staff members were observed for one period of duty each, 8 were on early duty and 4 on late duty, which was the average number of staff on each period of duty when the observations were made. Apart from the Ward Sister who was in charge when she was on duty only two other staff members were observed when they were in charge of the ward, both these occasions occurred on late duty. The Ward Sister or her deputy was observed on five occasions, three times on early duty and twice on late duty.

On night duty ten staff members were observed for one period of duty each. This number was greater than the average number of staff on duty but all the staff usually assigned to the ward were observed. Night duty staff were not always assigned to the same ward each night. Learners were not assigned to night duty.

As many of the day staff worked part time, the number of staffing hours available were not reflected in the number of staff on duty.

The time spent by the staff member under observation was categorised as time spent in Planned or Unplanned Activities or as Available Time. Available Time was defined as: time spent during working hours in activities which do not contribute to the care of the patients directly or indirectly. This category included time spent in unofficial breaks, time spent talking about personal affairs, time reading newspapers or magazines or watching television and the difference between the official working hours and the amount of time actually spent on duty.

The unplanned activities were further divided into:

Emergency Activities: Actions taken in a life-threatening situation or other situation affecting patient safety.

Between Activities: Stopping to think or changing location between activities or waiting a "reasonable" time before starting another activity.

Nursing Observations: Short observations of a patient, other than observations listed on the nursing care plan; on night duty time spent observing a whole room.

Communication: Any verbal communication pertaining to patients or directions for work other than report or rounds.

Personal Activities: Actions contributing to personal comfort or hygiene or checking duty rota.

Other Unplanned Activities: Unplanned activities not described elsewhere.

It might be thought that the spending of time by staff members in some of the activities in the category Available Time such as social conversations or unofficial coffee breaks, helps to ameliorate ward morale. However, as such activities were unofficial it was not accepted that the amount of time spent in these activities should be incorporated in the ultimate workload calculations. As this method of calculating workload allows time for unplanned activities and as changes may occur in the planned activities, some free time may occur; this free time might be used for the activities described under the category Available Time. Another way of incorporating time for unofficial breaks would be to allow a specific percentage of time for Personal Time and to incorporate this percentage into the calculation. As at present no such time appears to be permitted, it was not included in the method of calculation described in this study.

If the percentage of time spent in Planned and Unplanned Activities were calculated as a percentage of the total time, the Available Time would be perpetuated. Therefore, in this study, the percentages of time spent in Planned and Unplanned Activities were calculated as percentages of the total time spent in Planned and Unplanned Activities only, omitting the time spent in Available Time.

Factors Which Might be Expected to Affect the Amount of Time Spent in Planned Activities, Unplanned Activities and Available Time

Factors which might be expected to affect the amount of time spent in Planned Activities, Unplanned Activities and Available Time are:

1. The number of staff on duty in relation to the workload.
2. The grade of staff member being observed.
3. The effect on the staff of being observed.

The Number of Staff on Duty in Relation to the Workload

If the number of staffing hours available exceeded the workload and the Planned Activities were evenly distributed throughout the staff, two reactions might be expected to occur. First, the staff might spend more time in planned care by working more slowly and, therefore, there might be little effect on the percentage of time spent in Planned Activities. The extent of the effect might depend on the difference between the available staffing hours and the workload and on the speed at which the work was done. In this situation each staff member would probably have fewer planned activities assigned than she would if the available staffing hours and workload were equal. Thus, percentage of total time spent in planned activities would be decreased if the speed of working was not changed. Secondly, the staff might also spend more time in Available Time; therefore, the percentage of Planned and Unplanned time spent in Planned Activities would be higher than the percentage of total time which might minimise the effect of the overstaffing.

If the number of staffing hours available were less than the workload and the Planned Activities were evenly distributed throughout the

74

staff, the staff might work more quickly and thus there might be little effect on the percentage of time spent in Planned Activities. The extent of the effect might depend on the difference between the available staffing hours and the workload and the speed at which the work was done. Each staff member would have more Planned Activities assigned than if the available staffing hours and workload were equal, therefore, the percentage of total time spent in Planned Activities would be greater. In this situation some Unplanned Activities might be ignored, for example, a staff member might fail to respond to a patient's signal for attention. If such a situation occurred the percentage of time spent in Unplanned Activities would be decreased and the percentage of time in Planned Activities increased. It might be thought that when insufficient staff is available less time would be spent in Available Time. However, it is also possible that staff, when under pressure of work, need more breaks, in order to cope with the situation. Another reaction to insufficient staffing might be an increase in overtime work. The amount of overtime would be included in working hours when calculating the percentage of time in each type of activity. Thus, there would be no effect on the percentage of time spent in Planned and Unplanned Activities due to overtime.

Short-term effects on the percentages of time spent in Planned and Unplanned Activities could be overcome by calculating the mean. However, if either short staffing or overstaffing was a permanent feature, the percentages calculated might be affected as described which might in turn have the effect of perpetuating the existing situation. In order to measure the effect of staffing on the percentage of time spent in the various categories, this method would have to be repeated while controlling the staffing at different levels. As this control was not possible in this study, the staffing factor could have affected the results.

The Grade of Staff Member being Observed

It might be expected that different grades of staff might have different work assignments because of their different abilities. This situation might result in different grades of staff spending different amounts of time in Planned and Unplanned Activities; for example, the trained staff might be more apt to answer the telephone as they are better able to give information about a patient's condition; this activity might increase the amount of time spent by the trained staff in Unplanned Activities.

The Effect on the Staff of being Observed.

The staff might be expected to react in several ways to being observed. These ways were discussed earlier in this Chapter. The observations to determine the percentages of time spent in Planned and Unplanned Activities were directed at one individual for her complete working day; therefore, it might be expected that the reactions would be more marked than they appeared to have been when specific activities were observed. However, the permanent staff had already been under observation for six months and appeared to accept the presence of the observer. It was assumed, therefore, that there was little effect on the working patterns due to the observer's presence.

Time Spent in Planned and Unplanned Activities on Day and Night Duty

In order to determine the percentages of time spent in Planned and Unplanned Activities the following information was necessary:

the code number of the staff member under observation
the hours of duty of the staff member under observation
the number of staff on duty
the number of patients
the time an activity started
the time an activity stopped
the type of activity; planned, unplanned or available time
the total time taken for the activity
the date.

The form used for collecting this information is shown in Appendix 4.

When two activities occurred simultaneously, for example: communication during a bed bath, the on-going activity (the bath) was recorded as occurring, the secondary activity (communication) was not recorded. As communication is an activity which can occur simultaneously with another activity, the percentage of time spent in this activity may appear lower than would be expected.

After collection of the data the category Other Unplanned Activities was scrutinised and re-categorised as it appeared that some episodes might initially have been unsuitably categorised.

Ward Routine for Day Duty

The following is a general description of the routine on day duty of the ward observed.

07.30 hours	Rounds of patients by day charge nurse with night charge nurse.
	Prepare and serve breakfasts.
07.45	Report by day charge nurse to day staff.
08.00	Collect dirty dishes.
	Prepare for bathing.
08.15	Baths and treatments.

09.00–09.30	(First staff breakfast.)
09.30–10.00	(Second staff breakfast.)
10.00	Give baths.
	Distribute medications.
	Distribute drinking water and serve teas.
	Give mouth care.
10.00	Measure and record four-hourly and twice-daily temperatures, pulses and respirations.
	Clean locker tops.
12.00	Prepare for lunches.
	Serve patient lunches.
12.30	Give General Nursing Care.*
13.00–13.30	(First staff lunch.)
13.30–14.00	(Second staff lunch.)
14.00	Distribute medicines.
	Measure and record four-hourly and daily temperatures, pulses and respirations.
	Prepare tea.
14.30	Serve tea.
15.00	Give General Nursing Care.
16.00–16.15	(Staff tea.)
17.00	Give General Nursing Care, prepare for supper.
	Serve suppers.
18.00	Distribute medicines.
	Put some patients to bed.
19.00	Measure and record four-hourly and twice-daily temperatures, pulses and respirations.
	General Nursing Care.
19.00–19.30	(First staff meal.)
19.30–20.00	(Second staff meal.)
20.30	Start to settle patients.
	Prepare hot drinks.

In addition to these ward routines other regularly occurring events were:

Doctors rounds.

Visiting hours: Saturday and Sunday	14.30–15.30 hours
Tuesday	19.00–19.30 hours
Wednesday	14.30–15.30 hours
Thursday	19.00–19.30 hours

Games: arranged for the patients on Thursday afternoons.
In-service education classes: held for the learners every Tuesday.

---

*General Nursing Care was defined as: assisting patients with toileting and washing, giving appropriate back care and straightening of bedclothes.

The effect of this routine upon the workload pattern is illustrated in Figure 1, which shows the average number of minutes spent per staff member in Planned Activities, Unplanned Activities, Available Time and meal breaks for each half hour of the day shift. It can be seen that the pattern throughout the day shift is uneven. When the amount of time spent in Planned Activities tends to be large, the amount of time spent in Unplanned Activities tends to decrease. Available Time is spread throughout the day shift with the exception of from 08.00 hours to 09.30 hours during which period the amount of time spent in Planned Activities was at its greatest.

It is suggested that two reasons for the difference in the amount of time spent in Planned Activities between the morning and afternoon are the overlap in staff during the afternoon and an actual decrease in the amount of planned work to be done. There may be two reasons for this decrease: first, an understood regulation that all bathing and bedmaking must be completed in the morning and second because visiting hours are held from 14.30–15.30 hours on Wednesdays, Saturdays and Sundays.

Bathing or assisting patients with bathing generally took the most time per patient of any activity. As baths were all completed in the morning, the workload was comparatively heavy. This heavy workload was reflected in the high average percentage of time spent in Planned Activities during the period when bathing was done— 08.00–10.00 hours.

The Unplanned Activities which occurred between 07.00 and 10.00 hours tended to be in the category "Between Activities", that is, waiting while patients were on the commode or waiting for assistance. After 10.00 hours this type of activity continued but there was also an increase in the amount of "Communication" and in time spent with patients. These activities continued until 16.30 hours when the Unplanned Activities again tended to be in the category, "Between Activities". At 20.00 hours these again changed to activities involving patient contact.

Also during the overlap of early and late duty staff the average percentage of time spent in Available Time was generally higher than during the morning. Some of this time was accounted for by staff taking longer than the official time for meal breaks but the remaining time generally consisted of incidents of purposeless breaks in work. Such breaks may occur because there is no apparent work to be done. (This could also be because nurses are not encouraged to be self-directed.)

Some Planned Activities occur at relatively fixed times. These activities include serving meals, distributing medications and change of shift reports. Other Planned Activities, however, might be re-scheduled in order to help balance the workload between morning and afternoon; such activities would include activities directly affecting patients such

78

FIGURE 1.

Average Number of Minutes Spent per Staff Member in Planned Activities, Unplanned Activities, Available Time and Meal Breaks for each Half Hour of the Day Shift.

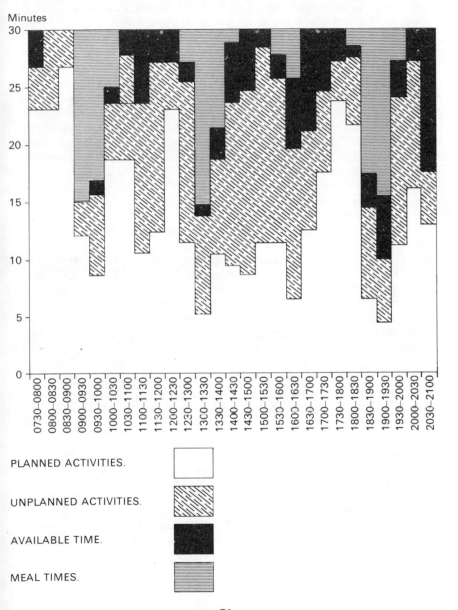

PLANNED ACTIVITIES.

UNPLANNED ACTIVITIES.

AVAILABLE TIME.

MEAL TIMES.

as the time when they are assisted with baths or have their beds made.

If Planned Activities were rescheduled so that the workload was more evenly distributed throughout the day shift the following might occur:

(a) Less time might be spent in Planned Activities in the morning and more time might be spent in Unplanned Activities.

(b) More time might be spent in Planned Activities in the afternoon and less time might be spent in Available Time.

(a) In the morning the average percentage of time spent in Planned Activities reached its peak and the average amount of time spent in Unplanned Activities was low. During this time the staff were involved with assisting patients with bathing and would be, therefore, with patients behind curtains or in the bathroom. Patients too would be behind curtains while dressing, therefore, not only would it be difficult for other patients to signal for attention, except by calling, but a staff member might be unable to leave the patient whom she was attending or might be out of hearing distance. The staff too would be unable to observe signs that patients required assistance—for example, a patient slipping from her chair.

If bathing activities were spread throughout the day, pressure to complete work by a certain time would be relieved and it is possible that the staff could then be accessible to attend to patients' impromptu needs.

The number of incidents of Unplanned Activities related directly to patients is considerably increased in the afternoon. This observation could occur because the patients are receiving less intensified personal attention than they might receive during a bathing session, the patients may, therefore, have more requests during the afternoon, and it may also be easier to attract the attention of the nursing staff. In the event that this assumption is correct the average amount of time spent in Unplanned Activities throughout the early shift would not be affected by rescheduling Planned Activities. If, however, the increase in Unplanned Activities during the afternoon arises because of an inability in the morning to intercept signals for attention then rescheduling Planned Activities might increase the number of Unplanned Activities which occur during the morning.

(b) If some of the time spent in Available Time occurs because there appears to be no work to be done, then be rescheduling some of the Planned Activities ot occur in the afternoon this problem might be alleviated.

If the workload was redistributed the average percentage of time spent in Planned Activities and Unplanned Activities might be affected. It is not expected that such a change would be great as the planned workload would not vary because of redistribution although the Unplanned workload might increase slightly. The average percentage of time spent in both Planned and Unplanned Activities might be affected by a change in the amount of time spent in Available Time.

Another method of dealing with the imbalance in the workload between morning and afternoon would be redistribution of staff to alleviate the overlap. This redistribution could be affected by a change to a three-shift system or by employing part-time staff to work during the morning period only.

There was also an imbalance in the average amount of time spent in Planned Activities during the evening period. This imbalance may be largely due to the staff's meal break when there may be insufficient staff on the ward to undertake any Planned Activities which require more than one person. Although two staff members may have been on the ward, if both became involved in care which required two people in one room, patients in other rooms would have been unobserved. Activities which required lifting of patients, therefore, had to be scheduled to occur when all staff members had returned from their meal. This problem would appear to be insoluble. Extra staff to relieve for meal breaks could not come from other wards where the problem would be similar. Extension of staff cafeteria hours so that only one staff member need be off the ward at one time might be of some assistance to the ward in question but would be of little help to smaller wards. Such an extension might create staffing problems in the Catering Department.

The average amount of time spent in Planned Activities fluctuated during the day duty shift. This fluctuation may have been due partly to the routine nature of the work. Some activities must be relatively routine such as serving meals to the patients, in order that the meal is served at a proper temperature. Such a routine probably requires concentration to the exclusion of most Unplanned Activities. However, other Planned Activities could perhaps be better spread throughout the day such as baths and bedmaking.

There was not the large decrease in the average amount of time spent in Planned Activities that might have been expected during the overlap of staff. The average number of minutes spent in Planned Activities between 07.45 hours and 12.00 hours was 18 minutes compared with 12 minutes between 12.00 hours and 16.30 hours. Between 16.30 hours and 21.00 hours this average was 15 minutes.

The fluctuation in the average number of minutes spent in Planned Activities per half hour was greater during the evening period possibly because during the evening meal break, when for one hour an average of only two staff were on duty, few Planned Activities could be scheduled.

Some fluctuation between Planned and Unplanned Activities is probably inevitable. If all the Planned Activities occurred at a fixed time and there was a large difference between the average percentage of time spent in Planned Activities at different periods during the day,

TABLE 4

Mean Percentages of Planned/Unplanned Time Spent in Planned and Unplanned Activities

	Number of Patients	Day of Week	Total Staff	Grade of Staff	Hours Worked	Staff in Charge Indicated by Asterisk	Planned and Unplanned Time		Percentage Total Time Available
							% Planned	% Unplanned	
0730–1630	26	Tues.	7	Aux.*	0730–1200		73	27	3
	22	Mon.	8	Aux.	0730–1530		90	10	30
	30	Wed.	7	RGN**	0730–1430		74	26	9
	30	Fri.	8	Pupil Nurse	0730–1630		83	17	19
	25	Wed.	7	Student Nurse	0730–1630		68	32	20
	26	Tues.	9	Enroll Nurse	0730–1630		57	43	7
	29	Fri.	6	Student Nurse	0730–1400		56	44	11
	32	Mon.	10	Aux.	0730–1630		73	27	14
1200–2100	27	Fri.	4	Aux.	1200–2100		78	22	36
	25	Tues.	4	Aux.	1630–2100		90	10	28
	26	Fri.	4	RGN	1200–2100	*	59	41	21
	23	Mon.	4	Student Nurse	1200–2100	*	72	28	12
Total							873	327	210
Mean							73%	27%	18%
Median							73	27	16.5
Standard Deviation							11	11	11

* Aux. Refers to a nursing auxiliary.
** RGN refers to a registered nurse.

82

then it would have been necessary to calculate different workloads and staffing levels required for those different periods. However, since the average percentages of time spent in Planned Activities did not change to a great extent during the day the day duty workload and required staffing could be calculated as a single entity. The overlap of staff would make it difficult to calculate the workload separately as both early and late staffs participated in the same activities and no activity which occurred during the overlap could be ascribed to either the early or late staffs.

Provided that there was sufficient staff on duty at any time to undertake the Planned Activities which must occur at that specific time such as serving meals and distributing medications, and provided that other Planned Activities were arranged to occur when the staff was on duty the workload could be undertaken at any period during the day shift. For example, baths which were usually done early in the morning might be done in the afternoon or evening if there were more staff on duty at these periods than early in the morning.

Table 4 illustrates the results of the individual calculations for day duty of the percentage of time spent in Planned and Unplanned Activities and the percentage of total time spent in "Available Time".

The average percentage of time spent in planned activities on day duty subsequently used in calculating the workload was 73%.

There did not appear to be any connection between the number of staff on duty and the percentage of time spent in Planned and Unplanned Activities, as illustrated in Table 5. However, the number of staff on duty does not correspond with the number of staffing hours available as many of the staff worked part time.

The percentage of time spent by each grade of staff in the three categories on day duty were compared (Table 6). On day duty the nursing auxiliaries spent an average of 81% of their time in Planned Activities and 19% in Unplanned Activities compared with an average of 63% in Planned Activities and 37% in Unplanned Activities for all trained staff and an average of 70% in Planned and 30% in Unplanned Activities by all learners. As 3 out of 5 of the auxiliaries and 2 out of 3 of the trained staff worked part time, the full time and part time staff were considered separately (Table 7). The full time staff spent an average of 70% in Planned Activities and 30% in Unplanned Activities compared with 77% and 23% respectively by the part time staff. The hours worked by the part time staff tended to be from 07.30 hours to 14.00 or 14.30 hours or from 16.30 hours to 21.00 hours. During most of these periods there is relatively less staff on duty as there is an overlap of the early and late staffs between noon and 16.30 hours except during meal breaks.

Therefore, when the part time staff are on duty, the amount of planned work for each staff member would be higher, which might cause the unplanned work to be decreased. However, as alluded to

TABLE 5

Percentages of Time spent in Planned and Unplanned Activities by All Staff except the Ward Sister Compared with the Number of Staff on Duty

Number of Staff	Percentage of Time Spent in Planned Activities	Percentage of Time Spent in Unplanned Activities	Total Percentage of Time Spent in Planned and Unplanned Activities
10	73	27	100
9	74	26	100
9	57	43	100
8	83	17	100
Mean	72	28	100
7	73	27	100
7	90	10	100
7	68	32	100
7	56	44	100
Mean	72	28	100

Because of the small numbers, the days when 10, 9 and 8 staff members were on duty were combined.

TABLE 6

Percentage of Time spent in Planned and Unplanned Activities on Day Duty by Various Grades of Staff

Staff	Number of Observations	Percentage of Time Spent in Planned Activities	Percentage of Time Spent in Unplanned Activities	Total %
Trained Staff	3	63	37	100
Learners	4	70	30	100
Nursing Auxiliaries	5	81	19	100

TABLE 7

Percentage of Time spent in Planned and Unplanned activities by Full and Part Time Staff

Staff	Number of Observations	Percentage of Time Spent in Planned Activities	Percentage of Time Spent in Unplanned Activities	Total %
Full Time	7	70	30	100
Part Time	5	77	23	100

earlier, in the morning, during the period when baths are given, staff may be behind curtains or in the bathroom with patients and, therefore, not available to undertake Unplanned Activities or there may be fewer patient initiated Unplanned Activities as patients' requests may be met during the bathing period. As it could not be determined whether the differences in the percentages of time spent in Planned and Unplanned Activities were due to the grade of staff or the Working hours, the mean percentages of time spent in Planned and Unplanned Activities were used in the calculation of workloads.

Ward Routine for Night Duty

There was no written routine for Planned Activities on night duty. The following list of night duty routines was based on observed practice.

20.45—On duty.
—Report.
21.00—Serve drinks to the patients.
—Four-hourly temperatures, pulses, respirations and blood pressures.
—Distribute medications.
22.00—Assist patients to bed.
—Give commodes/bedpans to Room 3.
23.00—Settle other patients for sleep.
—(First staff meal break.)
23.30—(Second staff meal break.)
00.00—Give commodes/bedpans to patients in Room 3.
—Distribute medications.
—Four-hourly temperatures, pulses, respirations and blood pressures.
02.00—Give commode/bedpans to patients in Room 3.
—Distribute medications.
03.00—(First staff meal break.)
03.30—(Second staff meal break.)
06.00—Give commodes/bedpans, assist patients out of bed, give basins to bedfast/chairfast patients.
—Distribute medications.
—Four-hourly temperatures, pulses, respirations and blood pressures.
07.00—Distribute cutlery to patients.
07.30—Report to day staff.

In addition to these activities the nurse in charge made rounds of the patients with the Night Sister or Nursing Officer who came to the ward three times during the shift. The nurse in charge was also responsible for recording the patients' conditions and preparing new pages for the patients' records.

The average number of minutes spent per staff per half hour in Planned Activities, General Observaion, Other Unplanned Activities and Available Time on night duty are illustrated in Figure 2.

It can be seen that the amount of time spent in Planned Activities was higher at the beginning and end of the shift and very low between 22.45–05.45 hours. The Planned Activities at the beginning of the shift, 20.45–22.45 hours consisted of: attending report, serving drinks, distributing medications, measuring temperatures, pulses and blood pressures and assisting patients to prepare for bed and sleep.

The Unplanned Activities during this period took little time and consisted mainly of attending to patients' needs.

A small amount of time was spent during this period in Available Time. The night duty staff reported to the Nursing Office for assignment to a ward and, therefore, did not arrive promptly on the ward at 20.45 hours. The rest of the Available Time was accounted for by unofficial breaks.

Between 22.45 and 05.45 the majority of the time was spent in General Observation. The small amount of time spent in Planned Activities during this period consisted of assisting patients with toileting and Rounds with the Night Sister.

The time spent in Unplanned Activities varied throughout this period and consisted mainly of attending to patients' requirements.

Available Time accounted for small amounts of time throughout the period.

Generally the morning "routine" started between 05.45–06.00 hours and from this period until 07.45 hours the amount of time spent in Planned Activities rose, the amount of time spent in Unplanned Activities decreased and no time was spent in General Observation. A small amount of time continued to be spent in Available Time.

As such differences in the amount of time spent in Planned Activities might affect the amount of staff required at various times throughout the night, the average percentages of time spent in Planned Activities, General Observation and other Unplanned Activities were calculated for the three different periods. These percentages are shown in Table 8.

It can be seen that the percentage of time spent in Planned Activities between 20.45–22.15 and 05.45–07.45 hours is considerably higher than between 22.15–05.45 hours. The percentage of time spent in General Observation was high between 22.15–05.45 hours. These findings reflect the pattern of work during the night. At the beginning of the shift treatments and measurements of vital signs might have been required, the patients would be assisted with toileting and preparing for bed; hence the large portion of time in Planned Activities. When the patients were in bed and sleeping, the amount of planned work to be done decreased. The planned work during this period included assisting with toileting, measurement of vital signs and administrative work. The majority of time when the patients were sleeping was spent

87

FIGURE 2.

Average Number of Minutes Spent per Half Hour in Planned Activities, General Observation, other Unplanned Activities and Meal Breaks during Night Duty.

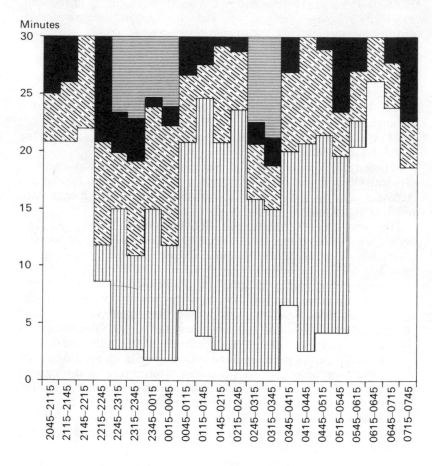

PLANNED ACTIVITIES.

GENERAL OBSERVATION

OTHER UNPLANNED ACTIVITIES.

AVAILABLE TIME.

MEAL BREAKS.

TABLE 8

Night Duty: Average Percentage of Planned Activities, Unplanned Activities, General Observation and Percentage of Total Time Spent in Available Time—for Three Periods

Time	Percentage of Time Spent in Planned Activities	Percentage of Time Spent in Unplanned Activities	Percentage of Time Spent in General Observation	Total	Percentage of Total Time Spent in Available Time
2045–2245	75	26	3	100	15
2246–0545	12	27	62	101	7
0546–0745	82	16	3	101	9

89

in observing for changes in the conditions of the patients and responding to patients' requests. An understood rule dictated that patients should not be wakened before 06.00 hours. The morning activities included wakening the patients, providing those who were not ambulant with a basin for washing, straightening bed clothes, arranging backrests and distributing place settings for breakfast. In order to complete these activities by the end of the shift, it is possible that patients' signals related to Unplanned Activities were not noticed by the staff, thus decreasing the time spent in Unplanned Activities. The number of other Unplanned Activities such as telephone calls, might be expected to be as great during this time as during the first two hours of the shift.

The 2% of total time spent in the category Available Time is, as would be expected, less than the average percentage of total time generally spent in that category. On five occasions no "Available Time" was recorded. This finding might also suggest pressure to complete the workload before finishing duty. Therefore, it is suggested that the average percentage of time used to calculate the workload at this time of day should be the same as that used for the first two hours of the shift. As there is only 1% difference between the average percentage of time spent in Planned Activities on day duty and that for the early part of night duty and the average of the two is 73%, it is suggested that the average percentage of time for Planned Activities for day duty and for the first and last two hours of night duty be taken as 73%.

As there appears to be a considerable difference between the amount of planned work to be done in the middle of the night and that at either end of the shift, it is suggested that ideally, the workload for these periods should be calculated separately. Separate calculation would be expected to indicate that the workload early in the morning is greater than the staffing hours which were available when the study was done. Possible methods of overcoming this difference in staffing hours and workload have been suggested in Chapter 4.

Because, on the ward observed, night duty was staffed as a continuous period of time, the average percentages of time spent in Planned and Unplanned Activities and General Observation for the complete shift were calculated. The results are shown in Table 9. For the purposes of this study, the average percentage of time spent in planned activities on night duty was accepted as 38%.

By calculating the workload on a single period rather than on three periods, the staffing during the first and last two hours of the shift might be slightly less than actually required and the staffing during the middle of the night higher than required according to the amount of planned activities to be done. However, there are other factors to be considered when calculating the amount of staff required on night duty such as the amount of General Observation to be done and the

TABLE 9

Night Duty: Measurements of the Percentages of Planned/Unplanned Time Spent in Planned Activities, Unplanned Activities, General Observation and Percentage of Total Time Spent in Available Time

No. of Patients	Day of Week	Total Staff	Grade of Staff	Staff in Charge Indicated by Asterisk	Percentage of Time Planned	Percentage of Time Unplanned	General Observations	Percentage of Total Available
25	Sun/Mon	4	Enroll	*	32	30	38	7
27	Mon/Tues	4	Aux.		38	21	41	9
24	Tues/Wed	4	Aux.		35	16	49	8
27	Wed/Thur	4	Enroll	*	45	13	43	9
38	Wed/Thur	4	Enroll	*	44	28	28	4
38	Thur/Fri	4	Aux.		35	32	33	10
39	Fri/Sat	4	Enroll	*	40	37	23	11
39	Sat/Sun	5	Aux.		33	26	41	19
39	Tues/Wed	4	Aux.		46	24	30	12
39	Wed/Thur	4	Aux.		35	23	42	9
Total					383	250	368	98
Mean					38%	25%	37%	10%
Median					36.5	25	39.5	9
Mode					35	–	–	9
Standard Deviation					4.91	6.88	7.62	3.71

coverage for meal breaks. Calculating the night duty workload as one period does not allow for the higher percentage of Planned Activities, lower percentage of Unplanned Activities early in the morning. Table 10 shows the calculations made for night duty staffing in two ways, considering the night as two periods and as one period. When the full time equivalent staff is calculated for the period 20.45 hours to 22.45 hours and 05.46 hours to 07.45 hours using 73% as the average percentage of time spent in Planned Activities, the full time equivalent

TABLE 10

Calculations for Night Duty Staffing

If the Amount of Planned Time between 20.45 and 07.45 is Taken as 1,000 Minutes:

From 20.45 to 22.45 and 05.46 to 07.45:
Average Percentage of Time for Planned Activities is 73%.
Therefore:

$73\% = 870$ Minutes (Amount of Time Required for Planned Activities)

$100\% = \dfrac{870 \times 100}{73}$

$= 1191.78$ Minutes

$= 19.86$ Hours

$= 4.97$ or 5 Full Time Equivalent Staff.

From 22.46 to 05.45:
Average Percentage Time Required for Planned Activities is 13%.
Therefore:

$13\% = 130$ Minutes (Amount of Time Required for Planned Activities)

$100\% = \dfrac{130 \times 100}{13}$

$= 1000$ Minutes

$= 16.67$ Hours

$= 2.78$ or 3 Full Time Equivalent Staff

From 20.45 to 07.45 (One Period)
Average Percentage of Time Required for Planned Activities if 38%
Therefore:

$38\% = 100$ Minutes (Amount of Time Required for Planned Activities)

$100\% = \dfrac{1000 \times 100}{38}$

$= 2631.58$ Minutes

$= 43.86$ Hours

$= 4.39$ or 4 Full Time Equivalent Staff.

92

staff required is 5. For the remaining part of the night, using 13% as the average percentage of time spent in Planned Activities the full time equivalent staff required is 3. This number of staff may be increased to cover for General Observation and staff meals. If the workload is calculated in one period using 38% as the average percentage of time spent in Planned Activities the full time equivalent staff required is 4. If the ward had 4 staff on duty for the eleven-hour night shift, the staff would either have to work more quickly to complete the work over the time span or concentrate on Planned Activities to the detriment of Unplanned Activities. However, if the ward had 5 staff on during the whole night, it might be overstaffed during the middle of that period unless 5 staff were required for General Observation.

With the exception of one day there were always four staff members on night duty. Therefore, no comparison could be made between the percentages of time spent in Planned and Unplanned Activities when the staffing was different.

The differences in the percentages of time spent by the trained and untrained staff in Planned and Unplanned Activities (excluding General Observation) was only 3% while in General Observation the difference was 6%. These findings are shown in Table 11.

No conclusions can be drawn from these small differences.

TABLE 11

Percentage of Time Spent in Planned Activities, General Observation and Other Unplanned Activities on Night Duty by Trained and Untrained Staff

Staff	Planned Activities	General Observation	Other Unplanned Activities
Trained	40	33	27
Untrained	37	39	24

The Ward Sister

It was suggested in Chapter 4 that part of the ward sister's functions are unique and, therefore, she cannot be equated to full time staff. The Ward Sister spent an average of 14% of her time in communication compared with an average of 4% by all other staff. This result would be expected as the Ward Sister was in charge when she was on duty, the nurse in charge for the other day period was only in charge when the Ward Sister was off duty. On the Ward Sister's day off the person in charge during the overlap of periods might have been determined by grade or seniority. This person would be in charge for the same length of time as the Ward Sister, if she were a full time staff member. Even in this situation, however, she has not the same authority as the Ward

93

Sister to make certain decisions, and, therefore, the percentage of time spent by the nurse in charge of the ward in communication might not be as high as that of the Ward Sister. The two nurses observed when they were in charge of the ward were both on the opposite period of duty from the Ward Sister and were, therefore, only actually in charge when she was off duty.

The average percentage of time spent by the Ward Sister in "Available Time" was 6% compared with 18% by all other staff. This finding may have been partly due to the fact that she usually undertook some work during her coffee/tea breaks.

The Ward Sister was the only person observed on day duty who spent time in the category "Emergency Activities". This emergency occurred in the evening when the Ward Sister was on duty with a student nurse in the third year of her training, a pupil nurse and a nursing axiliary and, therefore, the Ward Sister was the person mainly involved in attending to the patient. There did not appear to be a high incidence of emergencies on the ward.

The average percentage of time spent by the Ward Sister in all other categories was comparable with that spent by all other staff members excluding Planned Activities and Other Unplanned Activities. Both these categories would include Planned and Unplanned Activities related to the unique functions of the Ward Sister.

In order to calculate the percentage of her time required for her unique functions it would be necessary to know the optimum amounts of time which should be spent by Ward Sisters in various activities such as teaching and "carrying out nursing procedures and treatments", which would require a separate study. The amount of time actually spent by Ward Sisters in teaching should not be used as a

TABLE 12

Day Duty: Ward Sister, Percentage of Time Spent in Planned and Unplanned Activities.

Time on Duty	Percentage of Time In Planned Activities	Percentage of Time In Unplanned Activities	Total Percentage of Time Spent in Planned and Unlanned Activities
1200–2100	61	39	100
0730–1630	56	44	100
1200–2100	49	51	100
1200–2100	40	60	100
0730–1630	36	64	100
Mean	48	52	100
Median	49	51	100

basis for determining the amount of time Sisters should be given for teaching as it has been stated that this may be unsatisfactory (Chapter 4). Therefore, in this study, the percentage of time which the Ward Sister was to be allowed for her unique functions was calculated in the following way although it is recognised that it is not necessarily the optimum time.

As shown in Table 12, in five observations the Ward Sister spent an average of 48% of her time in Planned Activities. If her average is compared with the average which other staff members spent in Planned Activities, that is if the amount of time spent in Planned Activities is taken as 100%, then the time spent in Unplanned Activities stated as a percentage of the time spent in Planned Activities is 37% as shown in Figure 3.

FIGURE 3

Calculation of Unplanned Time Stated as a Percentage of Planned Time

If 73 = 100% of time spent in Planned Activities
then

$27 = \dfrac{100 \times 27}{73}\%$ of time spent in Planned Activities

= 37% of time spent in Planned Activities

If the Ward Sister is allocated 37% of the time which she spent in Planned Activities for Unplanned Activities, she is allocated 18% of her time for Unplanned Activities as shown in Figure 4.

FIGURE 4

Calculation of Percentage of Time Allocated To the Ward Sister for Unplanned Activities

If 100% of time spent in Planned Activities = 48
then 37% of time spent in Planned Activities = 18

If the Ward Sister spends 48% of her time in Planned Activities and 18% of her time in Unplanned Activities as performed by other staff members, she is left with 34% of her time for her unique functions. The Ward Sister could therefore be counted as being available for ordinary ward duties for five hours out of the eight hours that she is on duty or as .66 of a full time nurse.

Summary

In this chapter it was shown that the average percentage of time spent in Planned Activities on day duty by all staff excluding the Ward Sister was 73%. The Ward Sister cannot be equated to a full time staff member. Therefore, according to the amount of time spent in various activities by the Ward Sister observed, she should be calculated as .66 of a full time staff member. This policy leaves the remainder of her 8 hour day for her unique functions.

On night duty the average percentage of time spent in Planned Activities varied throughout the night. Therefore, ideally the workload should be calculated for different sections of the shift depending on the amount of Planned Activities usually scheduled. However, as ward staff were generally employed for the complete 11 hour shift, such calculations were impractical at this time. For this reason the night shift was treated as one unit. The average percentage of time spent in Planned Activities on night duty was 38%.

CHAPTER 8

Introduction and Operation
of the System
by the Researcher

The average percentage of time spent in Planned Activities on both day and night duty having been determined, it was considered essential to test the formula for calculating the workload.

It was decided that the researcher rather than the ward staff should transcribe the information required for the calculations. This practice would insure that the information was collected in the same way every day and there would be no need to teach several people how to do it. The motivation of the staff to collect information which had no immediate benefit to them would not affect the collection.

Although ideally the workload information should have been transcribed during the night in order that workload information could be available for the day shift, this practice would have been impractical as public transportation (which was not available during the night) had to be used by the researcher. Therefore it was decided that the information should be collected at 08.00 hours each morning.

As the researcher could not know the length of time required for the care of an individual patient, the trained ward staff were instructed in the recording of times on the nursing care plan. It was thought that this procedure would add only slightly to their workload. During the trial when times were not appended to the care described, the ward sister or nurse in charge was consulted or alternatively the average time for that activity was recorded.

The calculation of workload began on March 25, 1974 and ended on May 31, 1974. The information was recorded on three forms designed for this purpose. Sample completed pages are found in Appendices 5, 6 and 7.

The staffing hours were calculated to the nearest $\frac{1}{2}$ hour because the daily working time of some part time staff members included a $\frac{1}{2}$-hour unit (e.g. $5\frac{1}{2}$ hours). For day duty the full time staff was calculated to the nearest half as it seemed feasible to allow for half a working day of a full time staff member but not a smaller portion.

For night duty the staffing hours were also calculated to the nearest $\frac{1}{2}$ hour, but the full time staff numbers were calculated to the nearest whole as no staff members who worked less than 10 hours were employed on night duty.

In addition to calculating the staffing hours and full time staff required, the percentage of total time required for Planned Activities in each category was calculated.

Day Staffing

Appendix 8 illustrates the daily staffing hours and full time equivalent staff required on day duty. The staffing hours required on day duty ranged from 71 hours to 111 hours which corresponds to a range of full time equivalent staff of 9 to 14.

If the days are grouped according to the number of full time equivalent staff required on day duty, it can be seen in Table 13 that the average number of patients increased as the number of full time equivalent staff required increased which would suggest, not unexpectedly, that the number of full time equivalent staff required is to some extent related to the number of patients. However, this is not the only factor as the ranges overlap.

TABLE 13

Average Number of Patients on Days Requiring a Different Number of Staff

Number of staff required	Average number of patients	Range of number of patients
9	29	28–31
10	30	27–37
11	33	29–37
12	36	32–39
13	38	34–39
14	38	37–39

This ward required from 10 to 14 full time equivalent staff members on day duty on various days when the patient census was 37. Therefore other factors which might effect the number of full time equivalent staff required were explored. Table 14 shows the average number of full time staff required and the average number of minutes per patient required in each category according to the day of the week. The average number of patients varied by three with Thursday and Friday having the highest average number of patients at 35 and Sunday having the lowest at 32. The average number of full time staff ranged from 10 to 12 with Sunday requiring the lowest and Tuesday and Thursday the highest. On Tuesdays the average amount of time spent in "Rounds" was equal to the overall average, in "Meetings and Inservice Education" it was the highest. These two factors may have contributed to the need for more staff on Tuesdays. On Thursdays the average amount of time spent in "Rounds" was the highest. Thursday was one of two days when "Distraction Therapy" occurred. These may be two reasons in addition to the higher average number of patients for the higher requirement of staff.

The average amount of time spent in "Basic Care" and "Mobilisation" appeared to be unaffected by the day of the week. The average amount of time spent in "Technical Care" and "Individual Care" varied but there appeared to be no explanation related to the day of the week for the difference.

There was considerable difference in the average amount of time spent in "Observations" on Monday and that on other days. A possible explanation for this result was that those patients requiring weekly weight measurements were weighed on Monday.

The average amount of time spent in "Treatment by Medical Staff and/or Examination" was higher on Mondays and lower on Fridays,

TABLE 14

Average Number of Minutes Per Patient by Day of Week for Day Duty

Day	Mon.	Tues.	Wed.	Thurs.	Fri.	Sat.	Sun.
Average Number of Patients	33	33	33	35	35	34	32
Average Number of Staff Required	11	12	11	12	11	11	10
Basic Care	25	24	24	24	24	24	24
Mobilisation	26	26	26	25	25	25	27
Technical Care	2.7	3.6	3.0	2.8	3.5	3.7	2.9
Individual Care	4.7	4.6	4.3	4.3	4.8	4.6	5.2
Observation	10.5	8.4	8.1	8.4	8.2	8.2	8.0
Tests	1.3	1.0	1.0	.9	.5	.2	—
Future	1.6	1.0	1.1	1.1	1.5	1.1	.5
Report	4.9	5.2	5.0	5.0	4.6	4.2	4.5
Rounds	4.6	5.4	3.6	9.4	3.4	7.9	3.4
Administration	1.2	1.2	1.0	1.2	1.2	1.0	1.2
Medications	5.3	4.8	4.8	4.7	5.0	5.0	5.0
Housekeeping	2.6	2.5	2.6	2.4	2.5	2.5	2.6
Meals	27	27	27	27	27	27	27
Planned Admissions	.8	.5	.7	.5	.5	.3	—
Meetings	.6	7.9					
Distraction Therapy	5.6			5.2			

Saturdays and Sundays. The higher average on Mondays may be connected with the zero average on Sunday. It may have been that more specimens were collected on Mondays because laboratories were not open on Saturdays or Sundays. There was no apparent explanation for the Fridays results which was lower than all other weekdays.

Entries in the "Future" column related to discharges or arrangements for patients to leave the hospital for the weekend. There were fewer discharges on Sundays than any other day of the week and more on Monday and Fridays. It might be expected that patients would be discharged after the consultant's rounds but these differences in discharges did not seem to be related to consultant's rounds. The individual condition of each patient must have affected his/her discharge date. Therefore, although there were differences between the days, it is suggested that with the possible exception of Sundays, the day of the week was irrelevant.

Although there were differences in the daily average amounts of time spent in "Report", they could not be ascribed to the day of the week. The different number of staff on duty each day may have been one cause of the differences.

The average amount of time spent in "Rounds" varied each day due to doctor's rounds. The ward consultant held rounds on Tuesdays, Thursdays and Saturdays while other consultants who had patients on the ward held rounds on Mondays, Wednesdays and Fridays. Health team rounds were also held on Thursdays.

The average amount of time required for "Administration" was less on Wednesday and Saturdays as the pharmacy supplies were not checked on those days. There was no apparent explanation for the differences in the time required for "Medications".

The average amount of time per patient in "Housekeeping" and "Meals" was a fixed time and did not vary according to the day of the week.

The average amount of time spent in "Planned Admissions" was higher on Monday and Wednesdays than on Tuesdays, Thursdays and Fridays. There were few planned admissions on Saturdays, possibly because no tests, and/or examinations could be done until Monday. This situation does not explain the apparent lack of admissions on Sunday. Some differences in planned admissions may have been due to "waiting days" when any patient requiring emergency admission would be admitted; on these days no admissions would be scheduled.

An average of 75 minutes was spent in "Meetings and Inservice Education" on Mondays. Only 2 episodes contributed to this result, 30 minutes required for orientation and a 120-minute meeting. The average 260 minutes for "Meetings and Inservice Education" on Tuesdays resulted from classes held for learners. No other meetings or inservice education were planned.

"Distraction Therapy" was scheduled for every Monday and

100

Thursday with an average of 180 minutes for each day. No other distraction therapy was scheduled.

The average number of minutes per patient spent in each of the categories is shown in Appendix 9. The possible effect of one category on the workload may be illustrated for the category "Basic Care". The average number of minutes per patient per day required for Basic Care ranged from 19 to 28 minutes with an average of 24 minutes and a Standard Deviation of 2. Even a difference of 2 minutes per patient per day for an average of 32 patients equals 64 minutes for this one category of care. When all categories of care listed on the nursing care plan were considered together, the average number of minutes per patient per day ranged from 55 to 81 with an average of 68 and a Standard Deviation of 5. Table 15 shows the average number of minutes per patient required for all categories of care listed on the nursing care plan by day of week.

TABLE 15

Average Number of Minutes Per Patient Required for Care Listed on the Care Plan, by Day of Week, for April and May 1974.

Day	Mon.	Tues.	Wed.	Thurs.	Fri.	Sat.	Sun.
	67	62	59	59	55	63	64
	67	64	62	60	63	64	65
	70	64	65	63	65	64	66
Minutes	70	67	66	64	65	65	66
per	71	67	67	65	67	66	66
patient	71	69	67	65	69	68	68
	75	71	68	66	70	72	71
	75	75	71	70	72	73	73
	75	76	81	77	78		
Average	71	68 .	67	65	67	67	67

It can be seen that the average for Mondays was slightly higher than for other days of the week. This result could be due to the routine weighing of the patients who required weekly weight measurements on Mondays. The average amount of time required per patient for care listed on the nursing care plan on Thursdays was slightly lower than for the rest of the week; there was no apparent explanation for this difference.

It is inevitable that the number of staffing hours required will rarely correspond exactly with the staffing hours provided because nursing staff are employed to work a set number of hours. Therefore, some margin of extra/insufficient staffing hours must be allowed. For the purposes of this study this margin was set at $\pm$ 4 hours per shift because it appeared to be difficult to provide staffing hours in a smaller quantity than $\frac{1}{2}$ a working day. Taking this margin into consideration, on 18 days out of 61 the actual staffing hours were acceptable. On 8 days the actual staffing hours were greater than those required and on 35 days the actual staffing hours were less than those required. On 8 days the difference between the staffing provided and that required was -8 hours or less, on 18 days it was between -8 and -16 hours and on 9 days it was over -16 hours.

Night Staffing

The full time equivalent staff required on night duty was based on the calculation made according to the formula described in this study and not on the basis of the number of staff required to carry out General Observation. The number of staffing hours required ranged from 37 hours to 61 hours corresponding to 4 to 6 full time equivalent staff working a ten hour shift.

In calculating the required staffing hours on night duty the number of patients at 08.00 hours was changed by the addition of the number of planned admissions and the deletion of the number of planned discharges. If the number of patients at 08.00 hours on the following morning was taken as the number of patients that was actually on the ward during the night, this assumption would be correct unless there were admission or deaths during the night. Then, on 21 days the expected number of patients during the night was correct. On 29 days there were more patients than expected and on 10 days there were fewer patients than expected. An increase over the expected number of patients could be due to emergency admissions or cancelled discharges. The difference between the expected and actual number of patients ranged between 1 and 8. On 11 occasions there was a difference of 1 patient, on 7 occasions there was a difference of 2 patients, on 8 occasions there was a difference of 3 patients and on one occasion each there was a difference of 4, 5 and 8 patients. A decrease in the expected number of patients could be due to the unexpected discharges or deaths. On 5 occasions the difference between the expected and actual number of patients was 1, on three occasions it was 2 and on two occasions it was 3 patients. These differences would affect the workload and, therefore, for greater accuracy the information for calculating the night duty staffing should be collected in the evening.

Table 16 shows the number of actual and required staffing hours for night duty, for the days when the expected number of patients was equal to the number of patients on the ward at 07.30 hours of the next day.

On 9 out of 21 days the required staffing hours were within ± 4 hours of the actual staffing hours. On 8 days the required staffing hours

TABLE 16

Actual and Required Staffing Hours for Night Duty when the Expected
Number of Patients was Equal to the Actual Number of Patients

Date	Actual staffing hours	Required Staffing hours	Difference
April 1	50	51	−1
7	40	52	−12
12	40	51	−11
18	40	55.5	−15.5
21	40	54.5	−14.5
23	50	56	−6
27	40	57	−17
30	50	55.5	−5.5
May 5	50	48	+2
9	40	43	−3
13	40	40	—
17	50	51	−1
18	50	48	+2
19	50	41.5	+8.5
20	50	43	−7
21	50	43	+7
22	40	42	−2
24	50	45	+5
25	40	44	−4
26	40	42	−2
30	40	48	−8

were over 4 hours greater than the actual staffing hours and on 4 days the required staffing hours were over 4 hours less than the actual staffing hours. Table 17 shows the number of actual and required staffing hours for night duty for the days when the actual number of patients was less than that expected.

If the number of patients was less than expected the apparent under-staffing may not be as acute as demonstrated. As on 2 of these days the actual staffing had complied with the required staffing ±4 hours, this balance would have remained or the actual staffing hours would have been greater than those required. On the other 8 days it seems unlikely that the difference of 1 or 3 patients would have completely negated the difference between the actual and required staffing hours since few patients required 4 hours of care.

On 17 of these days the actual night duty staffing hours were below the required staffing hours for the expected number of patients; as any increase in the number of patients would cause some increase in the workload, these days would have a greater difference between the actual and required staffing hours. On 10 days the actual and required staffing hours would have balanced; however, with an addition of

TABLE 17
Actual and Required Staffing Hours for Night Duty when the Actual Number
of Patients was Less than the Expected Number of Patients

Date	Actual staffing hours	Required staffing hours	Difference	Difference between expected and actual number of patients
April 6	50	54	−4	−2
9	40	52.5	−12.5	−2
13	40	52	−12	−3
16	50	58	−8	−1
20	40	61	−21	−2
26	40	61.5	−21.5	−1
28	40	58	−18	−3
May 2	40	60	−20	−1
3	40	51	−11	−1
6	50	49	+1	−1

patients this balance may have been upset. On 2 days the actual
number of staffing hours was greater than those required by 7 and 9
hours. On these 2 days the number of patients was greater by 2 and 1
respectively, than those expected. Therefore, the actual staffing hours
may still have been greater than those required.

Therefore, it can be seen that on 33 out of 60 days the actual staffing
hours were less than the required staffing hours.

On day duty the average number of minutes per patient spent in
some categories was affected by the day of the week. As such a
difference could have an effect on the average number of staff required
on a particular day, the average number of minutes per patient on
night duty in the various categories was also examined.

Table 19 shows the average number of minutes spent per patient in
each category by day of week for night duty.

There were some differences in the average amount of time spent in
each category; none of these differences could be attributed to the day
of the week. The range of the daily average amount of time spent in
each category was:

Basic Care	.5–1.6 minutes
Mobilisation	15.8–22.8 minutes
Technical Care	.4– 6.3 minutes
Individual Care	0 – 1.1 minutes
Observations	1.2– 4.3 minutes
Treatments by doctors and/or Examinations	0 – 1.5 minutes

TABLE 18
Actual and Required Staffing Hours for Night Duty when the Actual Number
of Patients was Greater than the Expected Number of Patients

Date	Actual number of staffing hours	Required number of staffing hours	Difference	Difference between Expected and Actual number of patients
April 2	40	48.5	−8.5	+2
4	40	52.5	−12.5	+1
4	40	52	−12	+1
5	40	51	−11	+2
8	40	48	−8	+4
10	40	45.5	−5.5	+3
11	40	50	−10	+3
14	40	49	−9	+1
15	40	47	−7	+5
17	40	51	−11	+2
19	40	47	−7	+3
22	50	53.5	−3.5	+3
24	40	55	−15	+1
25	40	55	−15	+1
29	50	47.5	+2.5	+3
May 1	40	61	−21	+2
4	40	46	−6	+1
7	40	44	−4	+2
8	50	43	+7	+2
10	50	47	+3	+1
11	40	40	−	+1
12	50	41	+9	+1
14	40	40	−	+1
15	40	40	−	+2
16	40	44	−4	+3
23	40	42	−2	+3
27	30	37	−7	+3
28	30	39.5	−9.5	+1
29	40	43	−3	+8

The range in the number of full time equivalent staff required on both
day and night duty would appear to support the need for workloads
and staffing requirements to be calculated on a daily basis. In order to
accommodate for this daily fluctuation in ward staff it would seem
necessary to have some daily control over the assignment of staff
members. Such control may be exercised by re-assigning staff from
overstaffed wards to understaffed wards or by assigning pool staff to
understaffed wards.

TABLE 19
Average Number of Minutes Spent Per Patient in each Category by Day of
Week for Night Duty

Day	Mon./ Tues.	Tues./ Wed.	Wed./ Thurs.	Thurs./ Fri.	Fri./ Sat.	Sat./ Sun.	Sun./ Mon.
Average Number of Patients Expected	31	33	32	34	34	33	32
Basic Care	.9	.9	1.0	.9	.9	.9	.9
Mobilisation	19.8	19.2	19.3	18.8	18.9	19.4	20.3
Technical Care	1.3	1.9	1.6	1.4	2.1	2.5	1.7
Individual Care	.4	.5	.5	.5	.5	.5	.5
Observation	2.4	2.8	2.7	2.9	2.5	3.0	2.5
Tests	.7	.7	.6	.9	.6	.8	.6
Report	1.4	1.4	1.4	1.4	1.4	1.4	1.4
Rounds	.8	.8	.8	.8	.8	.8	.7
Administration	2.3	2.0	2.0	2.0	2.1	2.2	2.2
Meals	2.6	2.7	.26	2.6	2.6	2.7	2.7

In addition to the staffing hours required and the full time equivalent staff required, the percentage of time required for the whole day (24 hours) which was to be spent in each of the categories was calculated daily. It was believed that these figures would show any changes in practice on the ward and that the calculation of these percentages would, therefore, help to monitor such changes. The percentages should not be viewed in isolation but should be considered in conjunction with the number of hours which they represent. It was later decided that daily calculation was not required but that weekly figures would show any changes. The weekly average number of minutes and the average percentage of time spent in each category is illustrated in Appendix 10.

The average number of hours spent weekly in two categories "Distraction Therapy" and "Miscellaneous Preparation Time" remained constant but the average percentage of time in these two categories changed by .1 and .2% respectively as the total amount of time changed.

The average number of hours spent in all other categories changed. However, for "Individual Care", "Medications" and "Housekeeping" the average percentage of time did not change. This result was unexpected in the categories "Individual Care" and "Medications" as the activities in both these categories depend on the needs of individual patients. It was thought that, as the individual needs in these categories changed, the percentage of time would fluctuate. The average amount of time spent in "Housekeeping" varied by only 2 hours so the effect on the percentage of time was negligible.

The difference in the percentage of time spent in "Future", "Administration", "Planned Admissions" and "Meetings and Inservice Education" was also negligible.

The average difference in the percentage of time spent in other categories—"Basic Care", "Technical Care", "Observations", "Treatment by doctors and/or Examinations", "Report", "Rounds", and "Meals" varied by 1% or 2%. With this small range of average percentages of time spent in the categories, it would appear that these figures could be used as a base-line from which to measure changes.

Comparison of Results Using the Formula Described in this Study and the Aberdeen Formula[30,31] (Section I, Chapter 1)

A method of testing the suggested formula was to compare the results obtained by using the formula with those obtained by using another formula. It was not expected that the results would be the same as the basic assumptions of each formula are different, but the possible reasons for any difference may be considered.

The formula chosen for comparison was the "Aberdeen Formula". There were three reasons for this choice:

First: it required no additional work measurements on the part of the researcher. Some other methods of calculating workload or establishments might have involved additional time measurements. The "Aberdeen Formula" could be used to give crude results with the figures provided. Secondly: it was possible for the researcher to record the required information. Other possible formulae might have required recording by the ward staff which could have added to their workload. Thirdly: it was the formula which appeared to be best known and most likely to be used by nurse administrators in Scotland.

During the month of May 1974, daily information about the classification of patients according to the "Aberdeen Formula" was recorded. This information and the calculations are shown in Appendix 11. If according to that formula the allowed hours per week per patient were 20 hours, the following calculations can be made:

April/May 1974—average number of patients = 33
     multiplied by
     20 hours per patient $\underline{20}$
                         660 hours

660 hours divided by 40 hours per week
    per full time staff   = 16.5 full time staff

This figure can be compared with the calculations made according to the formula described in this study:

April/May 1974—number of staffing hours
required for day duty hours = 5469
divided by = 61 days
and multiplied by 7 days
628 days
628 hours divided by 40 hours per week = 16 full time staff
(15.7)

This is a difference of 32 hours or .8 of a full time staff member.

One apparent difference between the two methods is that the "Aberdeen Formula" operates on a retrospective basis whereas the suggested formula operates on a prospective basis.

It would have been desirable to compare the results reached daily by using each of the formulae. However, as the "Aberdeen Formula" was not meant to be used on a daily basis, such comparisons between the two formulae could not be made. However, as patients on the ward were categorising according to the "Aberdeen Formula" for four weeks in May 1974, weekly comparisons between the workloads calculated by using the two formulae can be made for this period (see Figure 5).

FIGURE 5

Weekly Staffing Hours Required as Calculated by the "Aberdeen Formula" and by the Formula Suggested in this Study

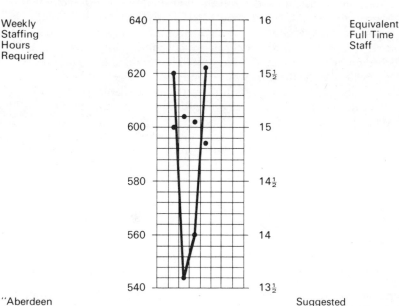

According to the "Aberdeen Formula", 15 full time staff members were required on each of the four weeks whereas according to the formula described in this study, the numbers of staff required over the four weeks were $15\frac{1}{2}$, $13\frac{1}{2}$, 14 and $15\frac{1}{2}$ respectively. Although these differences may appear to be negligible, at the least the difference is an average of almost 3 hours a day and at the most almost 9 hours a day or more than one full time staff member. The use of the "Aberdeen Formula" conceals the differences between days and, therefore, the discrepancies on specific days might be even more acute than is suggested by the averages.

Reasons for the differences in the required staffing hours using the two formulae are difficult to explain.

Although some of the category names in the two systems are identical, the items of care included under these categories differ. Also as the suggested system divides care in Planned and Unplanned Activities, direct comparisons of time spent in the categories cannot be made. Providing these differences are recognised some comparisons may be made. There may be a difference in the basic care given to each patient in the two systems; the "Aberdeen Formula" provides for a standard routine basic care for helpless patients, in the suggested formula the care is based upon the needs of each individual patient and even some helpless patients may not require the care described in the "Aberdeen Formula"; for example, certain patients may not require a daily bath.

The amount of time required for technical care in the suggested formula is considerably less than that allowed for in the "Aberdeen Formula", that is an average of 2 hours per patient per week of planned technical care compared with the fixed 4 hours per patient per week allowed in the "Aberdeen Formula" based on $47\frac{1}{2}\%$ of basic care required multiplied by average dependency. The ward observed in this study had several long-term patients awaiting geriatric placement; the technical care required by these patients may tend to be low and, therefore, to decrease the ward average.

Summary

The suggested system of calculating workload was carried out on one ward for two months. The number of full time equivalent staff required on day duty varied from 9 to 14. This result would support the need for daily workload calculations. Factors which appeared to affect the number of staff required were: the number of patients, the day of the week and the individual needs of the patients.

Other information such as the amount and percentage of time spent in various categories of care was also calculated. This information would be useful for making comparisons among wards and for determining changes in work patterns.

It was illustrated that the amount of staff required was affected by the day of the week. This information would be useful for planning duty rotas.

CHAPTER 9

Operation of the System
by the Ward Staff

As the system was only observed to have functioned when it was operated by the researcher, it was important to see if it could be operated by the ward staff because in actual use the ward staff would have to collect the information. Therefore, it was planned that with their permission the ward staff would participate in the system to the extent of entering times on the nursing care plans and transcribing the information during the night. The calculations would continue to be done by the researcher.

The Ward Sister was the first person from whom this permission was requested. If she refused there would have been no point in enquiring further. Having received the Ward Sister's approval, the Nursing Officer, Senior Nursing Officer, Night Nursing Officer and night duty staff were approached for their permission. In each case permission was granted.

The process of appending the amount of time required to the description of the care planned for each patient and described on the nursing care plan had to be explained to the new ward staff.

However, in practice, the researcher was not able to give instruction to the individual staff members because she felt that forcing the issue might have been unacceptable, thereby jeopardising the completion of the study.

The staff on night duty had to be instructed in the method of recording the information required. For this purpose it was necessary to redesign the second of the collection sheets as the ward staff were not as familiar with the information required as was the researcher.

In addition, a form on which to record actual staffing hours was introduced. Previously, the researcher had recorded this information on plain paper but a more detailed form was thought to be easier for the ward staff to use.

In order to assist the ward staff on both day and night duty in the operation of the system, a pamphlet containing the following information was supplied to the ward:

the instructions for inserting times on the nursing plans,
the instructions for completing the three pages of information
required to calculate the workload and a copy of each page,
a list of weekly routines,

111

a description of various activities and the average time required for each,

tables of various combinations of care related to "Mobilisation" and the average time for each section of the care and total average time required for the combination,

multiplication tables for various combinations of patients and/or staff.

In the period between the collection of workload information by the researcher and that by the ward staff there had been some changes to the ward. Two 8 bedded rooms on the second floor had been closed and the ward had become a 23 bed acute medical ward for female patients. This change had some effect on the workload apart from that caused by the reduction of the number of patients. For example, there was only one sluice to clean instead of two. The amount of time for "Rounds" and for serving meals was not changed despite the fact that these activities had formerly involved negotiating stairs, because any previous attempt had shown this time to be negligible. The time required for medicine rounds was not changed because the medicine trolley was still kept on the second floor and, therefore, the same amount of time was required for moving it to and from the first floor by lift.

Another change which occurred during the interim period was deletion of "checking pharmacy supplies" from the workload as this activity had been taken over by the pharmacists.

Because of the change in the number of beds and the other less important changes, it was expected that the results would be somewhat different from those obtained previously.

Collection of Information

The collection of information by the ward staff commenced on March 8, 1975. Some difficulties became apparent; these were:

the amount of time required for activities was not always entered on the nursing care plans,

page two of the collection forms was incorrectly completed as to the number of patients at various times throughout the day which changed due to expected admissions and discharges,

activities from the ward calendar which did not occur daily were not always recorded.

Because of these problems it was decided to reduce the number of entries required on the collection forms. This change made the forms easier to complete by making the calculations more complicated. A Busicom 207 calculator was available for use in the Nursing Research Unit. As a punch card programme could be employed for use in the calculator, the increased calculations could be done in a reasonable time. Previously the calculations of the time required for general ward activities were done individually. By using the Busicom calculator the fixed times could be included in the programme and only the variable numbers had to be entered; the multiplication and other calculations could be done automatically. Provision could be made for adding the number of admissions and subtracting the number of discharges from the number of patients. Because of this feature, the revised forms required the insertion of the number of patients at 03.00 hours only (the time during the night when the forms were most conveniently completed). The problem concerning the accuracy of the number of patients at various times throughout the day was thus removed. A programme for the calculation of workload was designed by the researcher for use with the Busicom 207.

Some of the other information which was omitted from the collecting sheets could be added by the researcher as it was generally information which was recorded in the ward diary. However, if no time was indicated on the nursing care plan or if no nursing care plan was initiated, there was no available information for the researcher to add.

During a period of time from March 8, 1975 to August 31, 1975 which covers 177 days, no information about the number of staffing hours available on day duty was recorded.

On 88 days there was insufficient information provided from which to calculate the staffing hours required for day duty; the same was true for 85 days in relation to night duty. On 28 days, 16% of the time, no information was recorded. The number of forms with insufficient information by day of week is shown in Table 20.

On 15 days, 80% of the time, the recordings were incomplete. On 9 of these days, the number of staff expected to come on duty was not recorded. Generally when this omission occurred the researcher was able to add the information. However, on a few occasions the forms were not collected daily and the missing information could not be added by the researcher.

On 45 days, 25% of the time, the times required for care was not recorded on the nursing care plans. This omission was usually indicated on the forms by the notation "no times stated" and occurred on week days rather than on the weekend when one of the nurses on night duty recorded the needed information on the nursing care plans. There was no obvious explanation for the higher incidence of missing times on Wednesdays shown in Table 20.

The Ward Sister felt that recording times on the nursing care plans took a considerable amount of her time. This comment suggested that the Ward Sister was the only member of the trained staff on day duty who recorded times on the nursing care plans. There may have been two reasons for the Ward Sister retaining this function. It may have been her preference to do so or the other trained staff members may have lacked the impetus or knowledge to record the times. As this

TABLE 20
Inadequately Completed Forms by Day of Week

Day of Week	Number of Days when			Total
	No Information Was Recorded	Other Information Missing	Times Not Recorded on Nursing Care Plan	
Monday	6	1	0	7
Tuesday	2	3	10	15
Wednesday	1	2	14	17
Thursday	6	3	11	20
Friday	8	1	10	18
Saturday	2	3	0	5
Sunday	3	2	0	5
Total	28	15	45	88

particular aspect accounted for the majority of days when the workload was not calculated, it must be considered in relation to the actual use of the system. It is suggested that in that situation all staff members would be instructed in the operation of the system. Therefore, the additional workload of appending times to the care described on the nursing care plans would be shared by all staff members. In fact, this recording could most easily be done at the time of describing care on the nursing care plan. It is suggested that if this work had been shared it would not have taken too much of one person's time.

In the actual use of this system workload information would be provided and used daily; therefore, the staff members would have greater motivation to record workload information and the work would have higher priority.

As the information required to calculate the workload was transcribed on 85 out of 177 days by the ward staff, it must be considered that there were no absolute difficulties which prevented the operation of the system by the ward staff.

The information recorded on the days when only partial information was given, was used in the calculations where possible, for example, in the calculations concerning particular categories of care.

Workload Information

In this section of the study it was important not only to determine if the ward staff could operate the system but also to continue to monitor the workload results.

The number of patients ranged from 15 to 23 with an average of 22 on the ward during this period (based on 155 days). The day staffing hours required ranged from 39.5 to 81 which equates to a full time staff of 5 to 10 (based on 85 days). Although the actual figures differ the range of staffing hours required on day duty for the two collection periods was within .5 hours. This result would support the argument that daily calculation of workloads is required.

On night duty the staffing hours required based only on workload figures and not on the staff required for General Observation, ranged from 17 to 53 which equates to 2 to 5 full time staff (based on 92 days). The range for staffing hours on night duty for the second collection period was greater (36) than for the first collection (25). Such a large difference could be due to the fact that there were more days in which the differences could occur. It also supports the need for daily calculation of the workload for night duty.

Summary

The ward staff undertook the operation of the system to calculate the workload to the extent which would be expected of staff in an actual situation. There were some problems with the collection of the information required for the calculations which might have been due to inadequate instruction or to the low priority which is naturally given to an unproductive project emanating from outside the hospital.

It appeared that the problems evidenced in this project were due to motivation and instruction rather than lack of capability. It is thought that if the staff members could see evidence of the effect of their efforts in a functioning system, such problems would be considerably lessened.

CHAPTER 10

Extension of the System to Other Areas

Although the system for calculating workload was seen to function on one ward, several points remained to be answered in relation to the introduction and operation of the system on a wider scale. Some factors which might affect the workload on different wards would be:

the physical structure of each ward,

the type of ward in relation to specialty,

the percentage of time spent in each ward in Planned and Unplanned Activities.

Any difference in structure of the ward would be incorporated in the amount of time required on each ward for various activities. Differences in practices related to Planned Activities would also be reflected in the system either by the inclusion of a specific activity or in the specific amount of time required for an activity by each ward. The amount of time spent in different categories such as "Basic Care" or "Technical Care" might be expected to differ among various types of wards in relation to specialty. Such differences may ultimately affect the percentages of time spent in Planned and Unplanned Activities. Conversely the different amounts of time required in various categories may balance each other and the percentages of time spent in planned activities remain roughly the same. The percentages of time spent in Planned and Unplanned Activities would be expected to be different on general and intensive care wards where, due to the acute conditions of the patients, the amount of time spent in Unplanned Activities would be expected to be higher.

If there are differences among wards in the percentages of time spent in Planned and Unplanned Activities, then comparisons between the amounts of time spent in various categories would be difficult. Comparisons of the amount of time required for any category would not reflect the percentage of time required and comparisons of the percentage of time required would not reflect the amount of time required. This difficulty might be overcome by comparing the percentages of planned time rather than percentages of total time.

In order to determine whether there was a difference in the percentages of time spent in Planned and Unplanned Activities on different types of wards, it was first necessary to determine if the percentages were the same on wards with the same medical specialty. Therefore, it was decided to expand the system into two other acute medical wards in the same hospital. These two wards, called Ward Two and Ward Three, were similar in physical structure to each other but were different from that on Ward One. Each ward contained three patient rooms of 8, 5 and 6 beds located on one floor. Ward Two was for male patients and Ward Three for female patients. The consultants and Nursing Officer were the same as on Ward One.

Permission for the expansion was sought and obtained from the Principal Nursing Officer, Senior Nursing Officer, Nursing Officers and Ward Sisters involved.

It was planned to send weekly reports of the daily workload information calculated to the Senior Nursing Officer, the day and night duty Nursing Officers and each Ward Sister. The system would run for six months after which a questionnaire about the collection of the information and the ultimate use to which it had been put would be distributed to the Senior Nursing Officer, the two Nursing Officers, the Ward Sisters and the night duty staff who took part in the collection.

The first step in the expansion was the calculation of the percentages of time spent in Planned and Unplanned Activities. The method used was the same as that for Ward One but fewer staff members were observed on each ward. Each staff member was asked individually for permission to be observed for the purpose of timing her activities. In each case permission was granted. On day duty on each ward, four staff members and the ward sister were observed on one period of duty each. The percentage of time spent in Planned and Unplanned Activities on day duty on both wards are shown in Table 21.

In the ultimate calculation the time spent in the category "Available Time" was again excluded.

The percentages of time spent in Planned and Unplanned Activities on night duty on both wards are shown in Table 22. Two staff members were observed on each ward, these were an enrolled nurse and a nursing assistant, the only other grade of staff which occasionally was on night duty was a registered nurse.

As these results were, with one exception, based on a small sample but were within the range of the results obtained on Ward One, the results from the three wards were combined and the mean of these results was used in the calculation of the workload on all three wards.

The average percentage of planned/unplanned time spent in Planned Activities used for calculating the workload for the day shift on the three wards was 70%. The average percentage of planned/unplanned time spent in Planned Activities used for calculating the workload for the night shift on the three wards was 38%.

Activities on Wards Two and Three were observed and timed on at least ten occasions. The time selected for use was the mode when one emerged, otherwise the mean was selected. These times were used either as fixed times in the case of general ward activities or as guidelines to assist the nurses in judging the amount of time required for individual patients. When activities did not occur frequently enough to obtain ten

TABLE 21

Percentages of Time Spent on Day Duty in Planned Activities, Unplanned Activities and Available Time on Wards 2 and 3

Ward 2				Excluding Available Time	
Staff Member Observed	Percentage of Time in Planned Activities	Percentage of Time in Unplanned Activities	Percentage of Available Time	Percentage of Time in Planned Activities	Percentage of Time in Unplanned Activities
Nursing Auxiliary on Early Duty	65	28	7	70	30
Pupil Nurse on Early Duty	72	22	7	77	23
Nursing Auxiliary on Late Duty	53	42	5	56	44
Student Nurse on Early Duty In Charge	64	30	6	68	32
Mean				68	32
Standard Deviation				7.57	

TABLE 21

Percentages of Time Spent on Day Duty in Planned Activities, Unplanned Activities and Available Time on Wards 2 and 3

Ward 3

Staff Member Observed	Percentage of Time in Planned Activities	Percentage of Time in Unplanned Activities	Percentage of Available Time		Percentage of Time in Planned Activities	Percentage of Time in Unplanned Activities
Registered Nurse on Late Duty	54	38	8		59	41
Enrolled Nurse on Early Duty	67	26	7		72	28
Enrolled Nurse on Late Duty	44	30	26		60	40
Registered Nurse on Late Duty	56	31	13		64	36
				Mean	64	36
			Standard Deviation		5.12	

119

TABLE 22

Percentages of Time Spent on Night Duty in Planned Activities, Unplanned Activities, General Observation and Available Time on Wards 2 and 3

Ward 2 Staff Member Observed	Percentage of Time in Planned Activities	Percentage of Time in Unplanned Activities	Percentage of Time in General Observation	Percentage of Available Time	Excluding Available Time		
					Percentage of Time in Planned Activities	Percentage of Time in Unplanned Activities	Percentage of Time in General Observation
Enrolled Nurse	44	19	36	1	45	19	36
Nursing Auxiliary	32	23	42	2	33	24	43
				Mean	39	22	40
Ward 3							
Enrolled Nurse	43	28	29	0	43	28	29
Nursing Auxiliary	25	25	46	4	26	26	48
				Mean	35	27	39

recordings, the observations made on all three wards were combined to obtain the mode or mean. This circumstance occurred only in the case of activities related to direct patient care and, therefore, would only be used as guidelines not as fixed times. The record of these observations are shown in Appendix 11.

Comparison of Time Required for Activities on Three Wards

Although it was expected that the average amounts of time required for activities on the three wards would not be the same there was one difference which illustrated the uniqueness of the wards. This was the amounts of time required for Reports, as illustrated in Table 23.

TABLE 23

Minutes Per Patient Required for Report of Three Wards

	Ward 1	Ward 2	Ward 3
Morning Report	.22	.70	.40
Noon Report	.40	1.70	1.0
Night Report	.30	.90	.60

Pamphlets which gave directions for the operation of the system including a list of the average times which had been obtained for each specific ward were given to the wards.

The ward staff members were instructed in the addition of the time required for activities listed on the nursing care plan. The night duty staff were instructed in the completion of the worksheets. The collection of workload information on the two new wards began on September 1, 1975 and was completed on February 28, 1976.

On all three wards there were occasions when the workload could not be calculated because the worksheets were not sufficiently completed. There were two main omissions, either no information was recorded or times were missing from some nursing care plans. Three had fewer admission due to the latter reason than did the other two wards. Otherwise the incidence was comparable.

As discussed previously these omissions could be due to pressure or work as the night staff were not permanently assigned to one ward, or lack of knowledge as to how to complete the worksheets. On Ward 1 worksheets were not completed most frequently on a Friday, on Wards 2 and 3 worksheets were not completed most frequently on a Monday.

There were also occasions when times were not listed on nursing care plans. This omission again did not occur on Saturday, Sunday or Monday on Ward 1, but was relatively evenly spaced throughout the week on Wards 2 and 3.

121

Occasionally on all three wards some information related to general ward activities was omitted from the forms.

The Required Staffing Hours on Three Wards

The ranges of staffing hours required on day duty for all three wards from September 1, 1975 to February 28, 1979 are shown in Table 24.

TABLE 24

Ranges of Staffing Hours Required on Day Duty on Three Wards From September 1, 1975 to February 28, 1976

	Ward 1	Ward 2	Ward 3
Range of Staffing Hours	41.5 —	37.5 —	58.5 —
Required	70.5	78	118
Average Staffing Hours Required	55	56	78.5

The ranges support the need for daily calculation of staffing hours.

If each ward has been provided with the average staffing hours required $\pm$ 4 hours, the comparisons between the available and required staffing hours would be as shown in Table 25.

TABLE 25

Comparison of Available and Required Staffing Hours for Day Duty on Three Wards if the Average Staffing Hours has been Provided

	Ward 1	Ward 2	Ward 3
Number of Days When	35	37	21
Staffing was Appropriate	44%	43%	18†
Number of Days of Over	22	26	54
Staffing	28%	30%	47%
Number of Days of Under	23	23	41
Staffing	29%	27%	35%
Total	80	86	116
	101%	100%	100%

On all three wards the number of days with adequate staffing hours was less than half of the days when the workload was calculated. It might be argued that the staffing hours available could be shared among the three wards as they were all acute medical wards. Therefore, the staffing hours required for one week on all three wards, shown in Table 26 was considered.

122

TABLE 26

Required and Available Staffing Hours on Day Duty for One Week, if the Average Staffing Hours had been Provided

Day	Mon.	Tues.	Wed.	Thur.	Fri.	Sat.	Sun.
Date	Dec. 1	Dec. 2	Dec. 3	Dec. 4	Dec. 5	Dec. 6	Dec. 7
Ward 1							
Required Staffing Hours	59	55	45	46	46	46	41
Available Staffing Hours	48	48	48	48	48	48	48
Difference	−11	−7	+3	+2	+2	+2	+7
Ward 2							
Required Staffing Hours		62	59	71	64	62	64
Available Staffing Hours		64	64	64	64	64	64
Difference		+2	+5	−7	−	+2	−
Ward 3							
Required Staffing Hours	60	61	53	46	49	51	51
Available Staffing Hours	53	53	53	53	53	53	53
Difference	−7	−8	−	+7	+4	+2	+2
Total Difference	−16	−13	+8	+2	+6	+6	+9

As can be seen in Table 26, on only one day, Thursday, would the extra staffing hours available on one ward cancel the deficit on another. On 4 days all the wards would have sufficient or extra staffing hours and on one day 2 wards would have insufficient staff which could not be supplied from the third ward. Therefore, it would seem that sharing of staff would not generally have been helpful.

Factors Affecting the Workload

In the first calculation the factors which were thought to effect the workload were: the number of patients, the day of the week and the care required by individual patients.

The Number of Patients

It can be seen from Table 27 that the ranges of staffing hours required for a certain patient census overlap.

TABLE 27

Ranges of Staffing Hours Required on Day Duty by Patient Census

Ward	Number of Patients	Range of Staffing Hours Required
1	18	41.5—41.5
	19	48 —55
	20	44 —60
	21	50 —62
	22	46 —65
	23	43 —70.5
2	15	42 —50
	16	40 —61
	17	37.5—67
	18	37.5—66
	19	48 —78
3	15	62 —71
	16	68 —79
	17	59 —92
	18	59 —107
	19	58.5—118

The upper limit of each range however, generally increases with the number of patients. These results would seem to support the premise that although the number of patients affects the number of staffing hours required to some extent, it is not the only factor involved. Some of the earlier methods of calculating nursing establishments alluded to in Chapter 1 were based on number of patients.

The Day of the Week

There were differences in the amounts of time required in some categories on certain days of the week. These differences varied among the wards and the majority were inexplicable. On Ward 3, for example, on day duty more time per patient was required for Basic Care on Mondays and Thursdays and less on Saturdays. The average minutes per patient by day of the week required in various categories is shown in Appendix 10.

The Care Required by Individual Patients

The care required by individual patients taken as a whole, that is the total of all care listed on the nursing care plans, required the largest amount of time in any category. Therefore, any changes in the amount of time required in this category would have a considerable effect on the staffing hours required. Tables 28 and 29 show the ranges in the number of minutes required on day and night duty for the total of the care required by individual patients.

124

TABLE 28

Ranges of Minutes Required for the Total Care Listed Daily on Nursing Care Plans for Day Duty

Ward	Range in Minutes	Difference in Hours
1	1061–1914	14
2	814–1950	19
3	1666–4164	41.6

TABLE 29

Ranges of Minutes Required for the Total Care Listed Daily on the Nursing Care Plans for Night Duty

Ward	Range in Minutes	Difference in Hours
1	425–1022	10
2	373– 538	6
3	538–1268	12

It is expected that these figures would be affected by the number of patients; therefore, it was important to consider the time required for care by individual patients. The number of minutes of care required by individual patients on day duty on Ward 2 as described on their nursing care plans ranged from 5 minutes to 489 minutes.

If groups of patients required the same care then it would be expected that there would be clustering around certain amounts of time required for care. There was no clustering but a mode of 15 minutes. The mode and other times which were required repeatedly were composed of times for different patients or for the same patient over a period of several days.

This wide range with no clustering and a progressive increase in time illustrates the effect that any one patient could have on the workload.

Fifty-seven per cent of the patients required one hour or less of planned direct care on day duty, 25% required from more than one hour up to three hours of care and 17% required between three and eight hours of care.

The Percentage of Time Spent in Various Categories

One of the benefits of producing information is the comparisons which can be made among wards. One of the factors which can be compared is the average percentage of time required for different categories.

Table 30 shows the average percentage of time spent in each category on each ward.

The average percentage of time spent in "Basic Care" was similar on all three wards for day duty but Ward 2 had a lower percentage required for night duty. A possible reason for this difference might be

125

TABLE 30

Average Percentage of Time Required in Each Category of Patient Care and General Ward Activities on Three Wards

| | Average Percentage of Time | | | | | |
| | Day Duty | | | Night Duty | | |
Category	Ward 1	Ward 2	Ward 3	Ward 1	Ward 2	Ward 3
Basic Care	17	17	16	8	5	8
Mobilisation	15	5	12	17	2	13
Technical Care	2	16	8	2	11	9
Individual Care	3	.1	13	.1	.1	.5
Observation	7	4	2	3	6	2
Treatment by Medical Staff and/or Investigation	—	—	—	—	—	—
Future	.2	.4	.1	—	—	—
Report	3	7	3	1.2	4	1.2
Rounds	4	4	3	15	2.2	1.0
Administration	.8	.7	.5	.9	1.3	.6
Medications	3	2	1	2	2	1
Housekeeping	1.5	.8	.6	—	—	—
Meals	13	12	8	3	2	1
Admissions	.1	.3	.1	—	—	—
Meetings and Inservice Education	—	—	—	—	—	—
Distraction Therapy	1	.0	.1	—	—	—
Miscellaneous Preparation Time	.5	.6	.4	.5	.8	.4
Total	71	71	68	39	37	38

the number of incontinent patients. Ward 2 had one long-term male patient who was occasionally incontinent whereas Wards 1 and 3 each had several long-term female patients who were incontinent.

The average percentage of time spent in "Mobilisation" on both day and night duty was much lower on Ward 2 than on the other two wards. Mobilisation and the toileting of patients are obviously related, as mobile patients can generally attend to their own toileting requirements. Female patients who require assistance with toileting may require bedpans or commodes, this is not true of male patients who use urinals for urination and require bedpans/commodes less frequently. The giving and removing of urinals takes much less time than the giving of a bedpan or commode. Ward 2 is a male ward, which may, therefore, account for the lower average percentage of time required for "Mobilisation".

There was no obvious explanation for the difference in the average percentage of time required for "Mobilisation" on Wards 1 and 3.

The average percentage of time required for "Technical Care" was very different on the three wards; there was no obvious explanation for these differences.

There was also a considerable difference in the three wards in the average percentage of time spent in "Individual Care" on day duty. This difference was expected as Ward 3 frequently had entries on the nursing care plans under this heading whereas this occurred only occasionally on Ward 1 but hardly ever on Ward 2.

Other inexplicable findings among the three wards were the differences in the average percentage of time required for Observation. As all wards were acute medical wards it was expected that the percentage of time spent in such activities as measuring temperatures and blood pressures would be similar.

The percentages of time required by all wards for "Treatments by the Medical Staff and/or Investigations" was very low, indeed for Ward 3 it was zero. It was expected that on medical wards the percentage of time required for this category would have been higher.

As the percentage of time required for the category "Future" generally would reflect the number of discharges it was expected that the percentages of time required would have been similar on the three wards, which was not the case.

The fixed time per patient for "Report" was different on each ward, therefore, it was expected that there would be a difference in the percentages of time required for this category. It was unexpected that Wards 1 and 3 had the same percentage.

As was expected the average percentage of time required for "Rounds" was similar on all three wards.

The average percentage of time required for "Administration" was very small and, therefore, more vulnerable to fluctuation due to differences in the amounts of time required for other categories. For this reason the small variation in the average percentages of time required in this category was insignificant.

The slightly higher average percentage of time required for "Medications" on Ward 1 may be due to the greater preparation time required because the trolley was kept on the second floor. Ward 1 also required a higher percentage of time for "Housekeeping" possibly also due to the longer preparation time.

There was no obvious reason for the average percentage of time required for "Meals" being lower on Ward 3 than on the other two wards. On night duty the higher percentage of time on Ward 1 may have been the result of the staff serving drinks whereas this task was undertaken by the day duty staff on the other wards.

The average percentage of time required for "Admissions" was almost negligible.

The average percentage of time required for "Meetings and Inservice Education" was higher on Ward 3. It appeared to the researcher that,

TABLE 31

Average Percentage of Time Required in Each Category by Month on Ward 3

Number of Days when Workload was Circulated		Sept. 25	Oct. 24	Nov. 30	Dec. 21	Jan. 24	Feb. 9
Basic Care	Day Duty	17	17	15	16	17	17
	Night Duty	8	9	8	7	7	7
Mobilisation	Day Duty	15	14	13	10	9	9
	Night Duty	17	15	15	10	9	8
Technical Care	Day Duty	4	6	5	11	11	14
	Night Duty	6	6	5	12	14	17
Individual Care	Day Duty	18	13	13	11	11	12
	Night Duty	1	.3	.4	.2	.6	0
Observation	Day Duty	1	2	2	2	2	1
	Night Duty	1	2	3	3	3	2
Treatment by Medical Staff and/or Investigation	Day Duty	0	0	.1	0	0	0
	Night Duty	0	0	0	0	0	0
Future	Day Duty	0	0	.1	.3	.2	.3
Report	Day Duty	2	3	3	3	3	3
	Night Duty	1	1	1	1	1	1

128

Category	Duty						
Rounds	Day Duty	3	3	3	3	3	2
	Night Duty	1	1	1	1	1	1
Administration	Day Duty	.5	.6	.5	.6	.5	.4
	Night Duty	.5	.6	.6	.8	.6	.6
Medications	Day Duty	1	2	1	2	1	1
	Night Duty	1	1	1	1	1	1
Housekeeping	Day Duty	.5	.6	.6	.6	.5	.4
Meals	Day Duty	8	9	9	9	8	7
	Night Duty	1	1	1	1	1	1
Admissions	Day Duty	0	0	0	0	0	.2
Meetings and Inservice Education	Day Duty	.4	.3	.8	3	2	.4
	Night Duty	0	0	0	0	0	.1
Distraction Therapy	Day Duty	0	0	0	.4	.2	0
Miscellaneous Preparation Time	Day Duty	.4	.4	.4	.5	.4	.3
	Night Duty	.3	.3	.4	.5	.4	.4
Total	Day Duty	70	68	69	70	71	69
Total	Night Duty	39	39	37	37	37	38

129

as the same Inservice Education opportunities were available to all wards, the difference could be due to a greater need for orientation.

Ward 1 had scheduled "Distraction Therapy" thrice weekly hence the higher average percentage of time for this category.

The different amounts and percentages of time required by the different wards in different categories demonstrates the individuality of the wards. Some of the difference occurred because of differences in the activities performed on the wards, for example the differences in "serving of night drinks". Others may be due to differences in the views of the nursing staff, for example the differences in the amounts of time required for "Individual Care" and "Distraction Therapy" and also the differences in the time required per patient for "Report".

It is possible that differences could occur due to failure to record care to be given, or other Planned Activities. In a working situation which was being monitored by the Nursing Officer, it is not thought that such omissions would be allowed to continue.

Another benefit of calculating the average percentages of time required for various categories is that changes can be monitored. Table 31 shows the monthly average percentage of time required for the categories of Care and General Ward Activities on Ward 3. There were several categories in which the average percentage of time required changed over the six months, these included "Mobilisation" on both day and night duty which dropped for the last three months. On the other hand the "Technical Care" required for those three months doubled. In retrospect the reasons for these changes could not be illustrated by the information collected; but would require immediate investigation in order to discover their causes.

The average percentage of time required for "Individual Care" was higher for September than for any other month. In September the staffing hours required on day duty on Ward 3 were considerably higher than the staffing hours available by an average of 39 hours or almost 5 full time equivalent staff. When the "Individual Care" was omitted from the calculation, the required staffing hours and the available staffing hours were more comparable. This result may have influenced the amount of time recorded for "Individual Care" on the patients' nursing care plans which did not contain a description of the particular care that was to be given.

The average percentage of time required for "Meetings and Inservice Education" was higher in October and November when two courses were held.

The Percentage of Time Spent by Ward Sisters in Planned Activities, Unplanned Activities and in their Unique Functions

It has been noted previously that the role of the Ward Sister is different from that of other nursing staff. For this reason the percentages of time spent by the Ward Sisters in Planned and Unplanned Activities were considered separately from those of the other staff members. The Ward Sisters spent less time in Planned Activities than did other staff. Table 32 illustrates the percentages of planned/unplanned time spent in Planned and Unplanned Activities and in work unique to the ward sister.

TABLE 32

Percentage of Time Spent in Planned and Unplanned Activities and in Work Unique to the Ward Sister

Planned Activities	Unplanned Activities	Unique to Sister	Total
50	39	12	101
56	29	15	100
49	36	14	99
40	50	10	100
36	51	13	100
53	33	14	100
44	50	6	100
47	41	12	Mean
49	39	13	Median
2.5	2.8	2.86	Standard Deviation

There may be several reasons for this result. Among the various categories of Unplanned Activities, the Ward Sisters spent more time in Communication" than did other staff members, 65 minutes compared with 20 minutes. This difference may be due to two factors: first that "Communication" was only indicated if no other activity occurred simultaneously. Therefore, many staff members may have communicated while continuing with another activity. The Ward Sister in her supervisory role may have moved from staff member to staff member to communicate with each and not have undertaken any other activity at the same time. Secondly, the Ward Sister may have been more in demand for communication as she was in a position to make certain decisions which other staff members would have to refer to her.

The Ward Sisters also spent a higher amount of time in the category "Other Unplanned Activities", 138 minutes compared with 95 minutes by other staff members. This difference may be due to the Ward Sister's position, she may be able to or be required to undertake certain activities. For example, as Ward Sister she would be ultimately responsible for maintaining emergency equipment in working order and would, therefore, be required to check such equipment. Although this is work which is known to have to be done, it does not usually have

131

a high priority and is made to fit in with other activities. Hence it is an Unplanned Activity.

The amount of time that Ward Sisters require to undertake their unique function has not been determined. In this study the average percentage of time spent by Ward Sisters in their unique functions was 12%. Whether this was sufficient time or not it is impossible to determine. Therefore, in order to determine the amount of time for which the Ward Sister might be attributed as being available to undertake the ordinary ward workload the following calculations might be made: if the workload is considered in terms of units and the total workload is equated to 100 units, then it could be said that ordinary staff members have 70 units of planned work to every 30 units of unplanned work. In addition to this the Ward Sister required an extra 19 units for unplanned work as Ward Sisters spent 19% more time in Unplanned Activities than did the average of other staff members and 12 units for unique work as they spent 12% of their time in their unique work.

Therefore:

70 units for planned work
30 units for unplanned work
19 units for extra unplanned work
12 units for unique work
—
131 units

As the ward sister works an 8-hour day—
131 units = 8 hours

$$1 \text{ unit} = \frac{8 \text{ hours}}{131}$$

70 units planned

$$= 100 \text{ units} = \frac{8 \times 100}{131} = 6 \text{ hours}$$

30 units unplanned

Therefore, the Ward Sister may be assumed as being available for 6 hours a day to undertake the calculated workload, which allows her 2 hours a day for her unique functions.

The figures used in this study were based on earlier calculations made after the observations on Ward One and described in Chapter 7. According to these calculations the Ward Sister was to be counted as available for general ward work for 5 hours a day.

Comparison of Time Taken for an Activity and the Time Listed on the Nursing Care Plan

As one of the problems of the system might be that the amount of time recorded on the nursing care plan could differ considerably from that actually taken, the following test procedure was implemented: the care given to a patient was observed and timed, and this measurement was compared with the care and time described on the nursing care plan. As the observation of the care of one patient might have involved a considerable period of time spent with little to observe, it was decided to observe two patients simultaneously. The first patient was selected at random and the second patient was the one to the immediate right of the first patient or if that bed was empty the second right, etc. In order to have observations covering the greater part of the working day of the patient the observations were made during the following time spans:

07.30 to 12.00 hours
12.00 to 16.30 hours
16.30 to 21.00 hours

As it was possible that the first patient might be moved in the ward, his care would continue to be observed over the three periods while the second patient would continue to be the patient to the right of the first patient. However, if the first patient was discharged the care given to the second patient would become the main focus of observation and the care of the patient to his right the second.

The activities observed generally came under the category headings "Basic Care" and "Observations". It was difficult to monitor the care listed under "Observations" as recordings may have been made just before or just after the observation period.

Omitting the partially observed "Observations", 8 activities took within one minute for brief activities and within 2 minutes for longer activities of the time listed on the nursing care plan. Three activities took less time than listed and 3 took more. It was difficult to make any judgment as to the accuracy of the times listed on the nursing care plans or to make any distinctions between the wards. Some of the activities which were not observed may have occurred at some other time or a decision may have been taken not to carry out certain care due to the condition of the patient. Another reason for the discrepancy may have been that the nursing care plans were out of date. In a working situation these problems would be overcome as one effect of out-of-date information might be insufficient staff and the possibility of this effect might encourage the updating of the nursing care plans.

Effect on the Workload of Changes Made on Nursing Care Plans During The Day

A factor which might affect the suitability of the staffing hours required as calculated by this system would be the difference in the time required which might occur due to changes in the care given to patients. In order to observe the effect of such changes a record of changes was made. Changes might be due to unexpected admissions

133

and/or discharges or to adjustments made in the care given to the patients. The time of day that such changes were made would to some extent determine the effect on the workload. However, it would be impossible without continuous observation to determine at what time the changes were made. As this study was carried out by one person continuous observation over the 24-hour period was not possible. Therefore, on the day of recording, entries or deletions on the nursing care plans of care to be given and the time required dated the previous day were noted. For example: on Ward One on December 19, 1975 two new orders were written. For one of these there was no time noted. The other required 44 minutes on day duty and 42 on night duty.

Because no time was indicated for many of the changes it was difficult to determine the extent of time change created by the amendments to the nursing care plans. On this ward the greatest change measured was due to an emergency admission. This type of activity was accommodated for by the time allowed for Unplanned Activities. The difference in the time recorded and the time subsequently applicable due to changes in the care given to patients on day duty ranged from 0 minutes to 307 minutes and for night duty from 0 minutes to 60 minutes. The mean of the actual changes on day duty (excluding days when there were no changes) was 43 minutes and the median 20 minutes. On night duty the mean 28 minutes and the median 24 minutes. There was only one day when the time change considerably exceeded the average. In such extreme circumstances the nursing officer should be made aware of the change in workload in order that she can take appropriate action. Apart from this one exception, differences in workload could be accommodated for by the time allowed for Unplanned Activities.

Views of Some Nursing Staff About the System of Calculating Workload

In order to ascertain from the nursing staff involved, their views about the method of collecting workload information, a small survey was conducted during February 1976, the last month of collection of workload information. A questionnaire was given to the Senior Nursing Officer, Nursing Officers and Ward Sisters who had received weekly workload/staffing information.

The purpose of this questionnaire was to ascertain what nurses in management positions thought about the workload information they had received and also to give them an opportunity to comment on this system of collecting workload data. Another purpose was to elicit from the Ward Sisters the amount of time required on the ward to operate the system. Six questionnaires were given to: one senior nursing officer, one nursing officer, one night duty nursing officer and three ward sisters. All six questionnaires were completed and returned. The responses were not separated by job category because of the small numbers. The questionnaire and covering letter sent to the management nurses are shown in Appendix 12.

The replies indicate that with a few reservations the information provided by this system although of little immediate benefit, might be useful in the future. Only one of the respondents would have liked daily information in order to make daily staffing arrangements. The nurses in management positions generally appeared to see the workload information in terms of long-term planning and not for deploying staff on a daily basis. This situation could have been influenced by the fact that they received information only once a week when they were unable to act on it.

Another questionnaire was given to staff members who participated in the study on night duty to elicit the amount of time required for completion of the worksheets and to ascertain what these nurses thought about the system. It was thought that such information might help to explain the apparent problems in operating the system, for example failure to complete all or part of the worksheets. Six questionnaires were given with envelopes in which they could be sealed and left for collection by the researcher. This questionnaire and covering letter are shown in Appendix 13.

One questionnaire was not answered, but a letter discussing the study was enclosed in the envelope.

The replies of the nurses would seem to indicate some difficulty with the medication portion of the worksheets. There does not appear to be any way of overcoming this difficulty with manual recording of the information. Computer application would eliminate this problem as the medications would already be recorded.

It was thought that seeing the results of their recording or non-recording might encourage the nurses to complete the worksheets. As apart from one nurse, generally they had not seen these results, this possible source of encouragement was lacking.

One factor mentioned by several of the night duty nurses was that frequently no times were appended to the care recorded on nursing care plans.

Overall the nursing care plan appeared to have made more impression on the night duty nursing staff than any other aspect of the study. This circumstance may have occurred because the nursing care plan was seen to be useful whereas the workload information may not have been seen as immediately of use.

The amount of time stated as required for the completion of the same worksheets ranged from 10 to 45 minutes with a mode of 30 minutes.

The amount of time expressed by the Ward Sisters as required to record the times required for activities on the nursing care plans varied. One Ward Sister was unable to comment, one suggested a total of 45

135

minutes inclusive for all staff and one a total of 70 inclusive minutes for all staff.

Summary

The system of calculating nursing workload was extended to two acute medical wards. The average percentage of time spent in Planned Activities on all three wards was similar so the "three ward" average of 70% was used for calculating all the workloads.

The working pattern of the three Ward Sisters was used to calculate the amount of time which Ward Sisters could be assumed to be available for general ward work which was 5 hours a day.

The workloads of the three wards were calculated over a period of 6 months during which time the results were sent to the Senior Nursing Officer, the Nursing Officer, the night duty Nursing Officer and the Ward Sisters. The opinions of the staff members involved in collecting the workload data and those who received them were elicited by means of a questionnaire.

An attempt was made to compare the time taken for an activity with the time listed on the nursing care plan. There were some discrepancies in these times but the reasons for them could not be ascertained.

The effect on the workload of changes made on nursing care plans during the day was measured and found, with one exception, that is, it could be accommodated for in the time allowed for Unplanned Activities.

SECTION III

CHAPTER 11

Summary, Recommendations and Conclusion

A method of calculating nursing workload based on individualised patient care has been described and tested. The researcher believes that any measurement of nursing workload should be based on the work that nurses should be doing rather than on what they are doing, as there are indications that there are differences between these two factors. The ideology of nursing accepted by the International Council of Nurses supports the idea of individualised patient care; it may be argued, therefore, that nurses should be giving individualised patient care and that the calculation of the nursing workload should be based on this tenet.

An aid to the practice of individualised patient care is the nursing care plan. A form for such a plan was designed and adopted for use in the group of hospitals where this study was carried out.

Some of the work done by nurses is planned, some unplanned. The amount of time required for the Planned Activities can be calculated. The amount of time required for Unplanned Activities cannot be calculated but the average percentage of time spent in both Planned and Unplanned Activities can be determined. If the amount of time required for Planned Activities and the average percentage of time spent in Planned Activities are known, the workload can be calculated using the formula:

$$\text{Workload} = \frac{\text{Amount of time required for Planned Activities}}{\text{Fraction of time spent in Planned Activities}}$$

The method of calculating nursing workload described in this thesis is based on individualised patient care. The benefits of such a system are:
(a) The information produced reflects immediately changes in the care given directly to patients,
(b) The information produced reflects immediately changes in general ward activities,
(c) The workloads for both day and night duty may be calculated,
(d) The collection of information does not add substantially to the workload of the nursing staff.

137

(a) The effects of care given directly to patients is immediately shown in the workload because the occurrence of activities related to care and the amount of time allocated for them are not fixed but reflect the actual daily schedule. Therefore, this system of calculating workload does not perpetuate a fixed routine or standard of care.

(b) General ward activities which occur other than daily would include Consultant's Rounds, Meetings and Inservice Education and Distraction Therapy. Although consultant's rounds may be scheduled to occur regularly, the routine can be changed; such a change would immediately be reflected in the workload calculations. Inservice Education sessions and Distraction Therapy sessions may also be regularly scheduled. However, in both these categories special events may be scheduled and by using the suggested method of calculating workload, the effect on the workload of such events would be immediately reflected.

(c) Most methods of calculating nursing workload which have been suggested are for day duty only. The method described in this study is suitable for both day and night duty workload calculations. The staffing required on night duty, however, should not be based only on the workload but also on the amount of General Observation required and the staffing required to provide coverage for staff meals.

(d) As the recording of a nursing care plan is seen by the researcher to be an integral part of nursing care it is not considered to cause an increase in the workload. The appending of times to the care described on the nursing care plan will add slightly to the workload. Any such increases in the workload may be justified by the improved information produced. The workload engendered by the processing of the workload would depend on the method of processing used. This factor would require consideration when discussing the feasibility of introducing the system.

In applying this system of calculating the nursing workload the commitment to the project of the nursing staff is an important factor as they would be responsible for recording the care required by patients, the amount of time required for this care and the general ward activities which are scheduled for a particular day. Non-commitment on the part of the nursing staff may create a problem as failure to record any one of these factors would make the calculated workload inaccurate.

The following factors might be considered in attempting to maximise the commitment of the nursing staff:

(i) adequate instruction of the nursing staff about the purpose and operation of the system,

(ii) support for the system by nursing administrators,

(iii) demonstration to the nursing staff that the information produced by the system is beneficial.

Preliminary Work to be Done Before the System can Become Operational

The following steps are necessary for the introduction of this system of calculating the nursing workload:

1. Determine the amount of time required for Planned Activities. This process is discussed in Section II, Chapter 6.

2. Determine the average percentage of time spent in Planned Activities for both shifts. This process is discussed in Section II, Chapter 7.

3. Append for each shift, the amount of time required to the care described on the nursing care plan.

4. Total for both shifts, the amounts of time listed on the nursing care plan and the amounts of time required for the general ward activities scheduled for that day, to give the total amount of time required for Planned Activities.

5. Calculate for both shifts, the total time required or workload on the basis of the total time required for Planned Activities equating to the average percentage of time required for Planned Activities.

6. Divide the workload by the number of hours worked daily on the relevant shift, to give the full time staff required.

7. Calculate the average percentage of time spent in the various categories of care and general ward activities.

In order to maintain the system re-timing of activities is required when changes are made in activities for which the time required was fixed. For example: if there was a change in the meal service, the time required for the newly defined activity would have to be measured.

Even when obvious changes do not occur activities may gradually be modified, so periodical reassessment of the fixed amounts of time required for activities would be desirable.

Comparison should also be made periodically of the amount of time required for activities which are based on nursing judgment and the actual time taken. This practice would assure the nursing officers that the nursing staff were not over-estimating the amount of time required and would serve to update the guidelines times as necessary.

Information Produced using this Method of Calculating Nursing Workload

The following information was produced using the method of calculating nursing workload described in this study:

1. The staffing hours and full time equivalent staff required on day and night duty.

2. The amount of time required daily by each patient for care described on the nursing care plan for both day and night duty.

Such information can be accumulated to show changes and trends and to give weekly, monthly or yearly totals for both individual wards and the entire hospital.

3. The weekly average percentage of time required in the various categories of care and general ward activities.

The ranges in the staffing hours required daily as shown in Tables 18 and 23 support the need for daily calculation of workload.

The ranges in the amount of time required for care for individual patients described on their nursing care plans, as shown in Table 39, supports the concept that the care required by individual patients affects the number of staffing hours required and that it should, therefore, be taken into consideration when calculating the workload.

Suggested Uses for the Information Produced

The workload information produced has several uses both short and long term, as described below.

Information about available and required staffing hours on various wards can be used by the Nursing Officer to re-deploy staff as necessary to reach a balance. She may be able to send to an understaffed ward, either a member of the pool staff or a nurse from an overstaffed ward. The Ward Sister will not need to make use of this information if the available and required staffing hours balance; however, if there are insufficient available staffing hours, the Ward Sister can determine the priorities in order to determine which activities should be discharged in the time available.

The Ward Sister or nurse in charge could use the information about the time required per patient for care described on the nursing care plan to assist in the allocation of care to be given.

The Ward Sister could use the accumulated information to determine if generally more or less staffing hours were required on certain days of the week and adjust her duty rota accordingly.

The average percentage of time required in each category of care and general ward activities illustrates the work done on a ward. The amount of time required in any one of the categories may be considered by the nursing officer to be too high or too low. Some of the categories to which this judgment might apply are: Report, Distraction Therapy, Meetings and Inservice Education. The amount of time required for these categories is based mostly upon the judgment of the nursing staff and is only slightly influenced by the number and condition of patients. Another category of care which might fit into this group is Individual Care. As the amount of time required in this category may depend on the opinions of the nursing staff about individualised patient care, an inappropriate requirement might indicate lack of knowledge about or disagreement with the concept of individualised patient care. In any of these instances, therefore, the nursing officer might wish to discuss the situation with the nursing staff.

Other categories of care and general ward activities are affected by the number and conditions of the patients or by other factors not easily

140

influenced by the nursing staff. Differences in the amount and percentages of time required in the categories of care and general ward activities on various wards might have a variety of causes; if the differences are not immediately explicable then the nursing officer may wish to investigate further the possible causes which might be management policies rather than be related to the type of ward.

Comparison could be made of the staff members on wards who spend different proportions of time in various categories. For example: the job satisfaction of staff members on wards where different percentages and amounts of time are required for Individual Care, Report and Inservice Education.

Information about the time and percentage of time required by the nursing staff to perform certain activities would be useful in discussions about the efficient performance of those tasks which lie within the grey area of responsibility between nursing and other staff. For example, in considering the serving of patients' meals the following factors may be considered:

(a) the amount of time required by nursing staff in serving meals and the cost of this time,

(b) the amount of time which would be required by other staff and the cost of this time,

(c) the activities which would be undertaken by the nursing staff if they were not serving meals,

(d) the activities performed by other staff members while the nursing staff are serving meals.

The nursing officer might also monitor exceptions from a set range of staffing hours required and exceptions from a range of average percentages of time required in categories of care. If the reasons for such exceptions are known they should be recorded, if they are unknown, the possible reasons for the exceptions should be investigated. This information could be used by nursing administrators in discussions about such changes with other departmental administrators; for example, the effect on nursing staffing requirements of an early discharge policy.

Senior nursing administrators could use the accumulated information on daily and weekly staffing requirements to assist in calculating the nursing establishments.

As the number of staffing hours varied from day to day on each ward consideration must be given to what the ward establishment should be and how to accommodate for discrepancies between the required and available staffing hours. Factors to be considered in calculating the establishment are: the number of full time staff required to execute the workload, the percentage of time allowed for sickness and the percentage of time allowed for holidays and vacation. Consideration might also be given to an allowance of time for Inservice Education and Research.

141

In this study the Ward Sister was adjudged as only a part of a full time staff member as she has certain unique functions, this factor must also be remembered when calculating the establishment. It has been suggested also that learners cannot be equated to full time staff; therefore, consideration should be given to the portion of a full time staff member with which a learner equates. These figures may depend on the experience of the learner.

The establishment may be divided into two sections, ward staff and pool staff. The ward establishment may consist of the average number of staff required on that ward. The pool staff establishment may consist of the remainder of the total establishment including the allowances for sickness, holidays, vacations, etc.

Pool staff are staff who may be assigned to any ward as they are not on the permanent establishment of a particular ward. If no pool staff is available the alternative system would allow for any staff member to be transferred temporarily to another ward. A disadvantage of this system is that staff members may resent moving to an unfamiliar ward. The experience of learners may be interrupted by transferring to another ward. On the other hand, if no suitable experience is available on the assigned ward another ward might be able to provide the necessary experience.

The pool staff may be comprised of part time, casual duty and temporary staff members. Using these staff members in this way may help to overcome any resentment on the part of full time staff members about having to work the hours and shifts rejected by part time or casual duty staff members.

Pool staff members may be assigned at the beginning of each period of duty according to the workload information on all wards received by nursing officers or they may be assigned for longer periods when a prolonged staffing shortage is foreseen.

Other Information Which Might be Provided Through the Suggested System of Calculating Nursing Workload

If this method of calculating nursing workload is operated manually the amount of information produced must necessarily be reduced as otherwise the work involved in producing the information might make the operation unfeasible. In order to produce the information suggested in the following paragraphs it is suggested that computerised nursing care plans would be required.

Whereas there are activities in nursing which can be undertaken only by trained staff there are few activities which should be only undertaken by untrained staff. The grade of staff required to undertake many activities depends on the condition of the patient. Therefore, it is important in calculating the staffing hours required on a ward to differentiate the grade of staff required. This was not done in this study

142

as it was important initially to ascertain that the basic system was workable. It is possible, however, using this system to determine the number of staff of the various grades required. This could be partially done by recording on the nursing care plan the lowest grade of staff required to undertake the activity for the individual patient. As there is an overlap of activities which may be performed by different grades of staff, noting the lowest grade of staff which can perform an activity provides for economic efficiency. The ratio of trained staff to learners must also be considered, as sufficient trained staff must be available to teach and supervise the work of learners.

If the required staffing hours could not be provided some decisions have to be made about the priority of the activities to be done. A comparison of the activities undertaken and those left undone in these circumstances would be useful in demonstrating the priorities which were set by the nursing staff and the effects of understaffing.

If understaffing were to remain a permanent feature, a list of the activities not being undertaken by the nursing staff would be useful in discussions about whether these activities were essential and if so what methods could be taken to ensure their execution.

In order to demonstrate which activities had not been done, it would be necessary to indicate which activities had been completed. A difficulty associated with this procedure might be resentment on behalf of the staff members about the monitoring of their work. Staff members might require assurance that the object of the procedure was to provide information about work which could not be completed because of ward circumstances rather than "checking up" on their work. A further difficulty might be recording as completed of activities which have not been undertaken. Part of the role of the ward sister is to supervise the work of her staff, therefore, she would in any case be monitoring the care given; this supervision would include the computerised recording as it now includes manual recording.

One of the items of information produced from this study was the amount of time required by individual patients for the care described on their nursing care plans. The number of patients who required 15 minutes or less of care on day duty was 13%. Such a small amount of care might include the making of the patient's bed and two or three Observations such as measurement of temperature, pulse and blood pressure. It would be of interest for the sake of the efficient use of hospitals to look further at the reasons why patients who require a very small amount of nursing care are in hospital.

In any study of nursing whether it be of quality care or patient outcomes, it would seem essential to know the staffing hours required and available, as any difference between these two could affect the situation being studied. Some of the studies which might be carried out using this information are:

(a) Comparison of patient outcomes on wards where the balance between required and available staffing hours is acceptable and wards with inappropriate staffing. Patient outcomes might include length of hospital stay, infection rate, satisfaction rate and incidence of postoperative vomiting. These outcomes are also influenced by other factors, however, as yet no effective method of measuring the effect of nursing care has been found.

(b) Comparison of staff turnover, illness rate and job satisfaction on wards where the balance between required and available staffing hours is acceptable and wards with inappropriate staffing.

The purpose of this research was to show a method of calculating the daily nursing workload. The operation of the workload was subsequently shown on three acute medical wards. Having accomplished that the next step would be to replicate the study in a larger area such as an entire hospital. Such a study would demonstrate whether the average percentage of time spent in Planned Activities could be generalised. The work necessary to calculate the workload for all the wards of a hospital would be considerable; it is, therefore, suggested that such a study would best be undertaken in a hospital using computerised nursing care plans.

This study was carried out in an acute general hospital. It is suggested, however, that this system is operable also in other types of hospitals such as hospitals for the mentally sub-normal, psychiatric hospitals and in the community. In any of these situations the care of patients requires planning and nursing care plans could be adapted for use. Some district nurses already use such a plan for the care of their patients.

It would seem advantageous to use the same method of calculating nursing workload for both the hospital and the community so that comparisons could be made.

Extension of the system to the community might prove uneconomic if nurses are practice based rather than geographically based unless a computer terminal was available in the practice offices.

Appendices

Nursing Care Plan and Rationale and Instructions For Its use

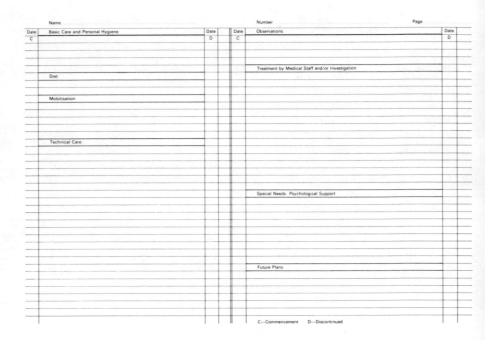

Name						Number		Page	
Date	Basic Care and Personal Hygiene		Date		Date	Observations			Date
C			D		C				D
						Treatment by Medical Staff and/or Investigation			
	Diet								
	Mobilisation								
	Technical Care								
						Special Needs Psychological Support			
						Future Plans			
						C—Commencement D—Discontinued			

A Nursing Care Plan is a written picture of the patient and his nursing care which enables the staff to give him the kind of care he has a right to receive.

PHILOSOPHY OF NURSING: W.H.O. Expert Committee on Nursing—Fifth Report.

Nursing Care: In a broad sense nursing care is derived from what has been called the unique function of the nurse. . .

> to assist the individual, sick or well, in the performance of those activities contributing to health or to recovery (or to peaceful death) that he would

perform unaided if he had the necessary strength, will or knowledge, and to do this in such a way as to help him gain independence as rapidly as possible. This aspect of her work, this part of her function, she initiates and controls: of this she is master.

Some of those activities for certain patients may be assigned by the nurse to less highly trained personnel under appropriate instruction and supervision.

If a patient's stay in hospital is achieved without loss of dignity, and if the patients are returned to their maximum function in the community, or are helped to a peaceful death, then the nurse's function has been fulfilled.

Roper, N. "Principles of Nursing" Second Edition, 1973.

Why a Nursing Care Plan?

To develop a more systematic way of thinking about and planning for individual patient care.

To provide a standard to assist student nurses to think logically in regard to patient care.

To provide a common pattern to facilitate orientation of student nurses around the group and the moving of all grades of staff between wards.

To establish, on the basis of the information provided about nursing care required, a nursing establishment.

Advantages:

It is a concise picture of a patient and his needs. Some of the information on the nursing care plan is presently available in other forms, i.e., bath book, ward diary.

The nursing care plan amalgamates this information and eliminates that need for re-writing it daily. It provides a structured form, uniform throughout the group of hospitals.

It provides a tool for expression of the philosophy of nursing.

It provides an extra method of communication for those small details about a patient which are not always passed on verbally.

It is also very useful for staff coming on duty at irregular hours.

Disadvantages:

It must be completely up to date to be useful and to avoid mistakes.

It could repress oral communication if allowed to do so.

Procedure for Use of The Nursing Care Plan:

A Nursing Care Plan, obtained from the stationery department, is initiated upon admission of a patient.

It is kept in the Kardex allotted for this purpose (may be separated from the Kardex) where it is retained until discharge, when it is filed with the patient's notes.

The nursing care is written in pencil by the member of staff admitting the patient. When the plans are approved by the nurse in charge they can be completed in ink.

The information on the cards should be checked during the reporting session but altered as appropriate throughout the day.

Guidelines for types of care which may be included under the following headings:

Basic Care and Personal Hygiene:

Type of bath, mouth care, skin care, dress required and if self care, part care, etc.

Diet

Mobilisation:

How to move the patient and maintain desirable posture, walking, sitting, lying and changing from one to another.

Technical Care:

Procedures to be done—dressings.

Procedures to be carried out by physiotherapists, speech therapists, occupational therapists, etc.

Investigations and/or Treatment by Medical Staff and Appointments:

Observations:

Temperature, pulse, respirations, weight, fluid balance, pupils, level of consciousness, etc.

Special Needs:

Under this heading the "special needs" of the patient should be identified and guidance should be given to indicate the physical and psychological support which the patient required.

The following aspects may be useful for the nurses to consider in planning how to help the patient:

(a) To avoid dangers to himself and avoid injuring others.

(b) To communicate his emotions, needs, fears, or feelings.

(c) To work at something which provides a sense of accomplishment.

(d) To play or participate in various forms of recreation.

(e) To learn, discover or satisfy curiosity that leads to "normal" development in health.

This help will range from cutting the patient's food, combing hair, etc., to listening and being aware of both physical and psychological needs. It will also entail support of relatives and friends.

Future Plans:

Discuss plans for rehabilitation, outpatient appointments, terminal care, education and instruction of both patient and/or family members, discharge and continuing care.

Measurement of Time Taken for Activities During One Period of Observation

Observation Number	Time	Staff Code	Description of Activity
8	1046	10	Turn on steriliser, upstairs for savlon—unable to find—back.
	1048	10	wash commodes
	1054		clear counter and scrub
	1057		wash incontinence pants
	1058		change dirty linen bags
	1058		finished downstairs sluice
9	1058	10	carry flowers into sluice—spill water
	1100		mop floor
	1100		get remaining flowers
	1103		carry flowers out to ward—return with trolley
	1104		away to help patient out of bed
	1106		clear trolley
	1106		back—clean emptied vases
	1107		for ward 2 flowers
	1110		out to ward
	1113		finished downstairs flowers
10	1238	1	rounds with doctor
	1306		away—back
	1325		rounds finished
11	1357	7	set up trolley—cups, milk
	1400		away—talking to sister
	1401	7	back—
	1402	7	away
	1421	7	back—kettle on waiting
	1425	7	back—check kettle, put on plates, make tea
	1429	7	away—bedpan

Observation Number	Time	Staff Code	Description of Activity
	1429	7	back—set out trolley—back to kitchen for saucers
		7	away—to help put patient back to bed
	1431	7	away—to help put patient back to bed
	1431	7	back
	1433	7	away—report
12	1420	7	sort menus
	1420		away
13	1434		afternoon report. 1 sister, 1 enrolled nurse, 1 pupil nurse, 1 nursing auxiliary
	1400		finished

Amounts of Time Determined for Planned Activities on Ward 1

Reports

Attending Morning Report: Given by Charge nurse on early day duty to the staff members on early day duty.	.3 minutes per patient
Making Rounds with night charge nurse: (first activity in the morning before report).	.22 minutes per patient
Attending Afternoon Report: given by early duty charge nurse to late shift staff members.	.4 minutes per patient
Attending Night Report: report by late duty charge nurse to night staff members.	.3 minutes per patient

Rounds

Making Rounds with Nursing Officer: by charge nurse.	.4 minutes per patient
Making Rounds with Consultant.	150 minutes*
Making Rounds with Registrar.	90 minutes*
Making Rounds with Health Team.	30 minutes*

Administration

Recording in the Kardex.	.75 minutes per patient
Preparing Evening Report for the Nursing Officer.	7 minutes*
Checking Pharmacy Supplies.	8 minutes*

Medications

Giving medications to patients.	1 minute per patient
Moving trolley.	12 minutes
Giving an injection: preparing, giving, recording and tidying.	6 minutes
Checking need for and giving aperients.	1 minute per patient

Housekeeping

Cleaning sluices: scrubbing bedpans and putting in steriliser, tidying sluice and cleaning draining board.	14 minutes

* Time determined on less than 10 observations and/or determined on the basis of discussion with the Ward Sister.

Cleaning locker tops: taking trolley around and washing all locker tops and overbed tables, replacing disposable bags on lockers.		1.5 minutes per patient
Setting up and cleaning trolley.		7 minutes
Waters: taking round trolley and distributing jugs and glasses to all patients unless fasting.		.4 minutes per patient

Meals and Drinks

Noon Meal: serving meals to patients.		9 minutes per patient
Evening meal: serving meals to patients.		11 minutes* per patient
Breakfast: preparing to serve meals	night duty	2 minutes
serving meals to patients	day staff	4 minutes*
	night duty	1.2 minutes* per patient
Menus: distributing menus for patients to complete, completing menus for those patients unable to do so.		.4 minutes* per patient
Teas: Making tea, setting up trolley with cups, feeders, milk, sugar, etc., returning trolley to kitchen, setting up lunch trolley with bowls, scoops, etc.		7 minutes
Serving tea.		1.2 minutes per patient
Evening drinks: Making tea, heating milk, setting up trolley for breakfast.		6 minutes*
Offering tea, cocoa, etc., to all patients.		1.5 minutes* per patient

Personal Hygiene

Big bath: including filling the bath, taking the patient to the bath, making the bed, dressing the patient and combing hair.		33 minutes
Big bath: including filling the bath, making the bed. Patient able to walk to bath but required some help.		25 minutes*
Make and open bed, with two staff.		8 minutes
Giving basin to patient who washes self in bed, making bed.		14 minutes
Bed Bath: Bathing a patient in bed, getting a patient up and making bed.		40 minutes
Bed bath: Bathing a patient in bed, making the bed with the patient in it.		33 minutes
Morning care: Assisting a patient with bedpan or commode, giving a patient a basin, straightening the bed clothes, rinsing dentures and combing hair.	1 staff	5 minutes
	2 staff	9 minutes
Straightening bed only.		2 minutes
Giving basin and straightening bed.		3 minutes

* Time determined on less than 10 observations and/or determined on the basis of discussion with the Ward Sister.

Hair Care

Washing, Setting and Drying a patient's hair		45 minutes*
Washing and Drying a patient's hair		16 minutes
Assisting a patient with bedpan or commode.	1 staff	4 minutes
	2 staff	6 minutes
Walking a patient to the bathroom.	1 staff	4 minutes
	2 staff	10 minutes
Changing an incontinent patient.		16 minutes
Put a patient to bed: patient able to get into bed without help. Putting in cradle if indicated, assisting with commode or bedpan.		5 minutes*
Lifting patient into bed after commode.		13 minutes*
Patient ambulant—preparing bed only.		1 minute
Settling a patient for sleep: lowering back	1 staff	1 minute
rest, putting in foot cradle if indicated.	2 staff	5 minutes
Feeding a patient: Breakfast or supper—2 courses		11 minutes
Noon meal—3 courses		20 minutes
Giving a drink to a patient.		4 minutes
Turning a patient, positioning and straightening bedclothes.		1 minute

Mouth Care

Using mouth care tray only.	4 minutes
Using mouth care tray and brushing dentures.	7 minutes*
Cleaning dentures and giving mouthwash to the patient.	3 minutes
Giving patient mouthwash only.	

Observations

Measuring and recording temperature, pulse and respiration.	5 minutes
Measuring and recording blood pressure.	3 minutes
Measuring and recording temperature and pulse.	3 minutes
Weighing a patient who requires help to get on the scales.	5 minutes
Weighing a patient who does not require help to get on the scales.	2 minutes

Admitting a patient

Filling in admission book, checking the patient's clothes. Putting the patient into bed if necessary and measuring temperature, pulse and respirations.	30 minutes

Discharging a patient

Includes helping the patient to pack, giving instructions for medications and return to clinic, stripping and washing the bed and locker and making the bed.	30 minutes*

Carrying out a Glucose Tolerance Test.

	30 minutes

* Time determined on less than 10 observations and/or determined on the basis of discussion with the Ward Sister.

Dressing a wound:

Includes setting up trolley, taking trolley to bedside, preparing   17 minutes*
the patient, washing, doing the dressing, returning and cleaning
the trolley.

Testing urine for sugar.   4 minutes

Giving a Wax Bath:

Includes transferring hot wax to container on trolley preparing   30 minutes*
towels, etc., taking to bedside, carrying out procedure,
returning wax and tidying trolley.

Attending a Ward Meeting.   35 minutes
                                                                     per staff
Attending Orientation to Ward.   15 minutes*
                                                                     per staff
Participating in Distraction Therapy.   30 minutes*
Monday and Thursday.   per staff

Miscellaneous Preparation Time.

Includes taking commodes, basins, linen,   Day Duty   23.5 minutes
trolley and laundry hamper into rooms
on routine rounds.   Night Duty   8 minutes

* Time determined on less than 10 observations and/or
determined on the basis of discussion with the Ward Sister.

Data Collecting Instrument for Recording the Amount of Time Spent in the categories Planned Activities, Unplanned Activities and Available Time

Date

Number of Patients:	Male	Female	Gynaecology
Number of Staff:	Sister (E)	Registered (E)	Student (E)
	(L)	Nurses (L)	Nurses (L)
	Enrolled (E)	Pupil (E)	Nursing (E)
	Nurses (L)	Nurses (L)	Auxiliaries (L)

Staff Number: (Period on Duty)

(E) = Early (L) = Late

Time		Unplanned Activities								Comment	Time
Start	Finish	Planned Activities	Emergency	Other Unplanned	Between Activities	Nursing Observation	Communication	Personal	Other		Total Minutes

APPENDIX 5

Direct Patient Care

Hospital   Ward   Date 5 April, 1974

Room	Bed	Basic Day	Basic Night	Mobilisation Day	Mobilisation Night	Technical care Day	Technical care Night	Individual Care Day	Individual Care Night	Observation Day	Observation Night	Tests Day	Tests Night	Future Day	Total
1	1	25	—	25	12					5					67
	2	25	—	20	11					5					61
	3	8	—	—	3					9	9				29
	4	8	—	—	3					15	5	5			36
	5	8	—	—	3	10				5					26
	6	43	6	15	3			28	4	13					112
	7	25			3					3					31
	8	25		50	28					5			5		113
2	1	40			3					20	10				73
	2	40		50	28					20	10				148
	3	61	8	76	43			30		3					221
	4	40			3					5					48
	5	33		56	42					30	15				176
	6	68	12	56	43	28	12	15		10					244
	7	40		21	17					29	16				123
3	1	15		20	11			15		6					67
	2	33		56	33			10		5					137
	3	15		26	26			40		14					121
	4	33		45	67			10							155
	5	33		81	67			15							196
	6	33		45	27			10							115
	7	33		61	53					3					150
	8	33			3									5	41

continued overleaf

157

| Patient | | Basic | | Mobilisation | | Technical care | | Individual Care | | Observation | | Tests | | Future | Total |
Room	Bed	Day	Night	Day	Night	Day	Night	Day	Night	Day	Night	Day	Night	Day	
4	1	8								10				30	48
	2	17	12	25	12					10					76
	3	40		21	17					20	10				108
	4	33		25	16					5					79
	5	8			3					3					14
	6	8			—					5					13
	7	8			3					5					16
	8	40		25	12					5					82
5	1	8								10		30		30	78
	2	25		10	3	5				7					50
	3	25								10				30	65
	4	8			3			32		3					46
	5	40		11	11					5					67
	6	33		11	12					20	10				86
	7	8			3					20	10	30			71
	8	33		25	16					32	15				121
Total		1059	38	856	643	33	22	205	4	375		60		90	4354

158

APPENDIX 6

General Ward Activities

Hospital   Ward   Date April 5, 1974.

Number of Staff. . . . . .Sister. . . . . . Late Duty
                                          Early.   7
                                          Late   3
                                          Night. . . . . .   (4)
Number of Patients   39

	Day	Night
Report		
Morning Rounds 39 × .22	8.58	8.58
Morning Report 39 × .3 × 7 + −.	81.9	—
Afternoon Report 37 × .4 × (4 + 1)	78	—
Night Report 37 × .3 × 4 (+1)	11.1	44.4
Rounds		
With Chief.	—	—
With Other Doctors	—	—
With Registrar	90	—
With Health Team	—	—
With Nursing Officer . . . Days 39 × .4	15.6	
Evenings 37 × .4	14.8	
10 p.m. 37 × .4		14.8
3 a.m. 37 × .4		14.8
6 a.m. 37 × .4		14.8
Administration		
Check Pharmacy Supplies	8	
Kardex . . . Day 39 × .75	29.25	
Night 37 × .75		27.75
Evening Report to Nursing Office.	7	
Medications		
Preparation (10 a.m. + Noon + 2 p.m. + 6 p.m.)	48	
Distribution: Patients on Medications (10 a.m. + noon + 2 p.m. + 6 p.m.) 76 × 1.	76	
Injections 2 × 6	12	12
Preparation (10 p.m. + 6 a.m.)	—	24
Distribution: Patients on Medications (10 p.m. + MN. + 2 a.m. + 6 a.m.) 46 × 1.		46
Aperiants 37 × 1.	37	

159

Housekeeping

Sluices   14
Lockers . . . Preparation   7
    Round 39×1.5 . . . .   58.7
Waters $39 \times .4$ 15.6

Meals

Breakfast 39×4   156
Dinner 39×9   351
Supper 37×11   429
Breakfast . . . Preparation   2
    37×1.2 . . . .   44.4
Distribute Menus $37 \times .4$ 14.8
Teas . . . 10 a.m. Preparation   7
    Serve 39×1.2 . . . .   46.8
   2 p.m. Preparation   7
    Serve 39×1.2 . . . .   46.8
   9 p.m. Preparation   6
    Serve 37×1.5 . . . .   55.5

Planned Admissions: 1×30   30

Meetings and Inservice Education

Ward Meeting $\times$ . . . .
Sister's Meeting . . . .
Unit Meeting . . . .
With Nursing Officer . . . .
With Nursing Officer . . . .
Committee . . . .
Orientation to Ward $+1 \times$ . . . .

Distraction Therapy

Bingo . . . No. of Staff $\times$ . . . .

_____ . . . .
_____ . . . .

Misc. Preparation Time . . . .

Other

_____ . . . .
_____ . . . .
_____ . . . .

Compilation Sheet

Hospital   Ward   Date

From Sheet One:	Day Total	Night Total	24 hr. Total	%
Basic Care	1059	38	1097	12%
Mobilisation	856	643	1499	17%
Technical Care	33	22	55	1%
Individual Care	205	4	209	2%
Observation	375	110	485	5%
Investigation, Treatment, Appointments	60	15	75	1%
Future	90	—	90	1%
From Sheet Two:				
Report	180	53	233	3%
Rounds	120	44	165	2%
Administration	44	28	72	1%
Medications	173	82	255	3%
Housekeeping	95	—	95	1%
Meals	1058	108	1166	13%
Planned Admissions	30	—	30	.3%
Meetings	—	—	—	—
Distraction Therapy	—	—	—	—
Misc. Preparation Time	23.5	8	31.5	.3%
Other				
Totals	4402	1156	5558	62.2%

To Calculate Ward Day Time Required: $\underline{A\ 4402} \times \dfrac{\underline{100}}{73} = \underline{6030}C$ Min.

$\quad$ C $\underline{6030}$ Min. + 60 = $\underline{100.5}$ D Hours

$\quad$ D $\underline{100.5}$ Hrs. + 8 = 12.56 Full Time Equivalent Staff

To Calculate Ward Night Time Required: $\underline{B\ 1156} + \dfrac{\underline{100}}{38} = 3042\,E$ Min.

$\quad$ E $\underline{3042}$ Min. + 60 = $\underline{50.7}\ F$ Hours

$\quad$ F $\underline{50.7}$ Hrs. + 10 = $\underline{5.07}$ Full Time Equivalent Staff

24 Hour Time = B $\underline{6030}$ + E $\underline{3042}$ = $\underline{9072}$ Min. = 60 = $\underline{151.2}$ Hrs.

Staffing Hours and Full Time Equivalent Staff Required for Day Duty April and May, 1974

Day	Date		Number of Patients at 8 a.m.	Staffing Hours Required	Full Time Equivalent Staff Required
Monday	April	1	39	108	14
Tuesday		2	38	102.5	13
Wednesday		3	39	99.5	12
Thursday		4	39	105	13
Friday		5	39	100.5	13
Saturday		6	39	99	12
Sunday		7	37	89	11
Total				703	
Average			39		12.5
Monday		8	37	99	12
Tuesday		9	37	99.5	12
Wednesday		10	34	82.5	10
Thursday		11	36	97	12
Friday		12	38	94.5	12
Saturday		13	37	98	12
Sunday		14	32	86	11
Total				656	
Average			36		11.5
Monday		15	33	97	12
Tuesday		16	37	111	14
Wednesday		17	35	93	12
Thursday		18	39	107.5	13
Friday		19	39	95.5	12
Saturday		20	39	105.5	13
Sunday		21	35	88.5	11
Total				698	
Average			37		12
Monday		22	35	102	13
Tuesday		23	38	104	13

Day	Date	Number of Patients at 8 a.m.	Staffing Hours Required	Full Time Equivalent Staff Required
Wednesday	24	38	101	13
Thursday	25	38	107	13
Friday	26	38	101.5	13
Saturday	27	37	95	12
Sunday	28	34	89	11
Total			699.5	
Average		37		12.5
Monday	April 29	32	89.5	11
Tuesday	30	32	98	12
Wednesday	May 1	32	93	12
Thursday	2	34	104.5	13
Friday	3	33	88	11
Saturday	4	32	83	10
Sunday	5	31	78.5	10
Total			634.5	
Average		32		11
Monday	6	31	90	11
Tuesday	7	31	82	10
Wednesday	8	31	74	9
Thursday	9	33	88	11
Friday	10	32	80.5	10
Saturday	11	29	75	9
Sunday	12	29	72	9
Total			561.5	
Average		31		10
Monday	13	28	78.5	10
Tuesday	14	28	77	10
Wednesday	15	28	70	9
Thursday	16	28	83	10
Friday	17	29	83	10
Saturday	18	30	83.5	10
Sunday	19	29	76	10
Total			551	
Average		29		10
Monday	20	28	82	10
Tuesday	21	28	82	10
Wednesday	22	29	74.5	9
Thursday	23	29	81.5	10
Friday	24	32	79	10
Saturday	25	30	78	10
Sunday	26	28	71	9
Total			548	
Average		29		10

Day	Date	Number of Patients at 8 a.m.	Staffing Hours Required	Full Time Equivalent Staff Required
Monday	27	27	78	10
Tuesday	28	29	84	11
Wednesday	28	29	84	11
Wednesday	29	30	76.5	10
Thursday	30	37	96.5	12
Friday	31	37	82	10
Total			417	
Average		32		11

Average Number of Minutes per Patient in Each Category of Care and General Ward Activities

	Day duty	Night duty
Basic Care	24	.9
Mobilisation	25	19
Technical Care	3	2
Individual Care	5	.5
Observation	9	3
Treatment by Medical Staff and/or Investigation	.7	.7
Future	1.1	—
Report	5	1.2
Administration	1.1	.7
Medications	5	2
Housekeeping	2.5	—
Meals	27	3
Admissions	.5	—
Meetings and Inservice Education	1	0
Distraction Therapy	1.6	.7
Miscellaneous Preparation Time	.7	
Medications	.24	

Average Number of Minutes Per Patient by Day of Week for Day Duty

Day	Mon.	Tues.	Wed.	Thurs.	Fri.	Sat.	Sun.
Average Number of Patients	33	33	33	35	35	34	32
Average Number of Staff Required	11	12	11	12	11	11	10
Basic Care	25	24	24	24	24	24	24
Mobilisation	26	26	26	25	25	25	27
Technical Care	2.7	3.6	3.0	2.8	3.5	3.7	2.9
Individual Care	4.7	4.6	4.3	4.3	4.8	4.6	5.2
Observation	10.5	8.4	8.1	8.4	8.2	8.2	8.0
Tests	1.3	1.0	1.0	.9	.5	.2	—
Future	1.6	1.0	1.1	1.1	1.5	1.1	.5
Report	4.9	5.2	5.0	5.0	4.6	4.2	4.5
Rounds	4.6	5.4	3.6	9.4	3.4	7.9	3.4
Administration	1.2	1.2	1.0	1.2	1.2	1.0	1.2
Medications	5.3	4.8	4.8	4.7	5.0	5.0	5.0
Housekeeping	2.6	2.5	2.6	2.4	2.5	2.5	2.6
Meals	27	27	27	27	27	27	27
Planned Admissions	.8	.5	.7	.5	.5	.3	—
Meetings	.6	7.9					
Distraction Therapy	5.6			5.2			

Classification of Patients According to the Aberdeen Formula and Calculations of the Staffing Hours Required Per Patient Per Week

The figures used for the basic nursing hours per week per equivalent patient, percentage technical nursing care required, hours per week per actual patient for administration and domestic activities, the percentage of time for miscellaneous activities and dependency factors were the updated figures for 1975.
Produced by one Scottish Health Board.

WORK SHEET FOR ABERDEEN FORMULA

Classification	A	B	C	D	E
1	2	4	9	7	10
2	2	5	9	9	9
3	2	5	11	4	11
4	2	11	5	3	11
5	1	10	3	5	12
6	1	9	5	5	11
7	1	10	5	3	11
8	1	6	7	2	14
9	1	7	7	5	13
10	1	8	7	3	12
11	2	8	6	4	9
12	2	10	6	4	8
13	1	11	6	4	6
14	1	10	7	3	7
15	1	10	7	3	7
16	1	11	7	3	5
17	2	12	9	3	3
18	2	12	7	4	5
19	2	13	7	3	5
20	1	13	7	3	4

Classification	A	B	C	D	E	
21	1	13	7	3	4	
22	1	12	7	3	6	
23	1	11	8	3	6	
24	1	11	8	3	10	
25	1	13	6	3	7	
26	1	11	7	3	6	
27	1	11	7	3	5	
28	1	11	9	3	4	
(b) Total for Period	36	278	186	104	221	
(c) Average for Period	1.28	9.93	6.64	3.71	7.89	29.45 Total
(d) Category Factor	1	.85	.75	.30	.25	
(e) Equivalent	1.28	8.44	4.98	1.11	1.97	17.78 Total

Dependency Factor $= \dfrac{\text{Total Col. (e) } 18}{\text{Total Col. (c) } 30} = .6$

Allowed Hrs./Wk. per actual patient =

Basic Nursing Hrs./Wk. + Technical Nursing × Average +
per Eq. Patient (M or F) (47½) Dependency
(14.45 + 6.84 × .6) +
Hrs./Wk. per Actual Patient Misc.
Admin. and Domestic + 6 3/4 = 20 Hrs.
4.75 + 1.25 +   1.29

Questionnaire and Covering Letter Given to Nurses in Management Positions

Department of Nursing Studies,
Nursing Research Unit,
12 Buccleuch Place,
Edinburgh,
January 27, 1976.

Dear

As the collection of data is due to stop on February 29, 1976 I would like to take this opportunity to thank you and your staff for the help and co-operation received over these past months. It has been a pleasure to work with all the staff.

I have another favour to ask of you; attached is a questionnaire which I would like you to complete. The instructions are on the form. A questionnaire has also been given to the night staff which they have been asked to leave on the ward for collection.

Thank you for your help.

Yours sincerely,

Confidential

Return to N. Grant,
Nursing Research Unit,
University of Edinburgh
12 Buccleuch Place,
Edinburgh

A METHOD OF CALCULATING A NURSING ESTABLISHMENT BASED ON INDIVIDUALISED PATIENT CARE.

QUESTIONNAIRE

Before the completion of this present phase of the research I would appreciate your opinion on certain points. Due to the small numbers of people involved anonymity cannot be assured but names will not be recorded. Please do not sign the form but post it in the attached envelope no later than February 15, 1979. Thank you.

1. Have you been able to make any use of the information provided for you?
Yes   No
If yes, in what way?

2. Can you think of any other ways in which this information might be used?
Yes   No
If yes, please describe it (them).

3a. Is there any other relevant information that you would have liked?
Yes   No
If yes, what is the information and how would it have been used?

3b. Is there any information provided that you consider to be superfluous?
Yes   No
If yes, what is it?

4. Would you find it helpful if the information had been provided daily?
Yes   No
If yes, what ways might it have been used?

5. Are you aware of any effects good or bad in the ward situation resulting from this research? Please tell me what they are:
Good effects:

Bad effects:

6. The collection of this type of information is bound to be time-consuming for the staff providing it. Do you feel that the time required for this method is excessive? Yes   No
Are there any other inconveniences associated with this method?
Yes   No
If yes, what are they?

7. Up to this point you have been asked specific questions, are there any comments you would like to make about the method of collecting and providing information about staffing or about the presence of a researcher on the wards? Please use this space overleaf if necessary.

8. WARD SISTERS ONLY
How long, on average, does it take, each day, for the day staff to record the time required for the activities listed on the nursing care plan? Ward Sister   Staff Nurse
Student/pupil nurse

170

Questionnaire and Covering Letter Given to Night Duty Nurses

Department of Nursing Studies,
Nursing Research Unit,
12 Buccleuch Place,
Edinburgh
January 27, 1976.

Dear

As the collection of data is due to stop on February 29, 1976, I would like to take this opportunity to thank you for your help and co-operation in collecting this information for me. You may feel that your contribution has been insignificant but your participation has been essential in showing how the system works at ward level.

I have one last favour to ask. Attached is a questionnaire which I would like you to complete; instructions are on the form. Thank you again.

Yours sincerely,

Confidential

Return to N. Grant,
Nursing Research Unit,
12 Buccleuch Place,
Edinburgh

A METHOD OF CALCULATING A NURSING ESTABLISHMENT BASED ON INDIVIDUALISED PATIENT CARE

QUESTIONNAIRE

Before the completion of this present part of the research I would appreciate your opinion on certain points, as you have been closely involved with the collection of information.

This questionnaire is anonymous although the ward is recorded. Please do not sign the form but seal it in the envelope provided no later than February 15, 1976. It will be collected from the ward. Thank you.

1. How much time, on average is required each day to complete the worksheets?

2. Is there anything which would make the worksheets easier for you to complete? Yes　　No

If yes, please tell me about it.

3. Were there any difficulties you had in assisting with this research? Yes　　No

If yes, please tell me about them.

4a. Have you seen the information on staffing returned to the ward weekly?
　Weekly　　Occasionally　　Never

4b. If you have seen it can you suggest ways in which this information might be used? Please tell me about them.

5. Are you aware of any effect good or bad on your work situation which this research has caused? Please tell me what they are:

Good effects:

Bad effects:

6. Up to now you have answered my questions; please use this space to add your own comments and observations.

References

1. DEPARTMENT OF HEALTH AND SOCIAL SECURITY, SCOTTISH HOME AND HEALTH DEPARTMENT AND WELSH OFFICE (1972). *Report of the Committee on Nursing*, p. 130. London: HMSO. Cmnd. 5115.
2. THE NUFFIELD PROVINCIAL HOSPITALS TRUST (1953). *The Work of Nurses in Hospital Wards. Report of a Job-Analysis*. London: The Nuffield Provincial Hospitals Trust.
3. LEEDS REGIONAL HOSPITAL BOARD (1963). *Work Measurement as a Basis for Calculating Nursing Establishment*. Leeds: Leeds Regional Hospital Board.
4. OPERATIONAL RESEARCH UNIT, OXFORD REGIONAL HOSPITAL BOARD (1967). *Measurement of Nursing Care*, No. 9. Oxford: Oxford Regional Hospital Board.
5. WORK STUDY DEPARTMENT, NORTH EASTERN REGIONAL HOSPITAL BOARD, SCOTLAND (1967). *Nursing Workload as a Basis for Staffing*. Scottish Health Service Studies No. 3. Edinburgh: Scottish Home and Health Department.
6. WORK STUDY DEPARTMENT, NORTH EASTERN REGIONAL HOSPITAL BOARD, SCOTLAND (1969). *Nursing Workload Per Patient as a Basis for Staffing*. Scottish Health Service Studies No. 9. Edinburgh: Scottish Home and Health Department.
7. HEARN, C. R. (1974). Evaluation of Patient's Nursing Needs: Prediction of Staffing 1, 2, 3, 4. *Nursing Times*, Vol. 70, pp. 69–84. (Occasional Papers.)
8. AULD, M. (1974). *A Method of Estimating the Requisite Nursing Establishments*. M. Phil. Thesis, University of Edinburgh. (Unpublished.)
9. DEPARTMENT OF HEALTH AND SOCIAL SECURITY, SCOTTISH HOME AND HEALTH DEPARTMENT AND WELSH OFFICE (1972). *Report of the Committee on Nursing*, p. 138. London: HMSO. Cmnd. 5115.
10. NURSING TIMES' EDITORIAL (1973). An Ostrich Attitude. *Nursing Times*, Vol. 69, No. 36, p. 1139.
11. DEPARTMENT OF HEALTH AND SOCIAL SECURITY, SCOTTISH HOME AND HEALTH DEPARTMENT AND WELSH OFFICE (1972). *Report of the Committee on Nursing* p. 20. London: HMSO. Cmnd. 5115.
12. IBID., p. 118.
13. THE SCOTSMAN (1973). Nursing: A Suitable Case for Treatment. *The Scotsman*, Nov. 6, 1973.
14. NURSING TIMES (1975). Fully Understaffed. *Nursing Times*, Vol. 71, No. 42, p. 1637.
15. DEPARTMENT OF HEALTH AND SOCIAL SECURITY, SCOTTISH HOME AND HEALTH DEPARTMENT AND WELSH OFFICE (1972). *Report of the Committee on Nursing*, pp. 131–2. London: HMSO. Cmnd. 5115.
16. LEEDS REGIONAL HOSPITAL BOARD (1963). *Work Measurement as a Basis for Calculating Nursing Establishments*, p. 3. Leeds: Leeds Regional Hospital Board.

17. KING EDWARD'S HOSPITAL FUND FOR LONDON (1945). *Considerations of Standards of Staffing.* Cited by: the Nuffield Provincial Hospitals Trust (1953). *The Work of Nurses In Hospital Wards,* p. 106. London: The Nuffield Provincial Hospitals Trust.

18. NURSING MIRROR (1975). Probe to Match Nurses with Needs. *Nursing Mirror,* Vol. 141, No. 22, p. 35.

19. LEEDS REGIONAL HOSPITAL BOARD (1963). *Work Measurement as a Basis for Calculating Nursing Establishments,* p. 59. Leeds: Leeds Regional Hospital Board.

20. THE NUFFIELD PROVINCIAL HOSPITALS TRUST (1953). *The Work of Nurses in Hospital Wards. Report of a Job Analysis,* pp. 41–2. London: The Nuffield Provincial Hospitals Trust.

21. IBID., p. 151.

22. LEEDS REGIONAL HOSPITAL BOARD (1963). *Work Measurement as a Basis for Calculating Nursing Establishments.* Leeds: Leeds Regional Hospital Board.

23. IBID., p. 7.

24. IBID., p. 57.

25. WOLFE, H. & YOUNG, J. P. (1963). Staffing the Nursing Unit: Part one: Controlled Variable Staffing. *Nursing Research,* Vol. 14, p. 237.

26. OPERATIONAL RESEARCH UNIT, OXFORD REGIONAL HOSPITAL BOARD (1967). *Measurement of Nursing Care.* No. 9. Oxford: Oxford Regional Hospital Board.

27. NORWICH, H. S. and SENIOR, O. E. (1971). Determining Nursing Establishment. *Nursing Times.* Vol. 67, No. 5, pp. 17–20. (Occasional Papers.)

28. MULLIGAN, B. (1972). How Many Nurses Equal Enough? *Nursing Times.* Vol. 68, No. 15, pp. 428–30.

29. WORK STUDY DEPARTMENT, NORTH EASTERN REGIONAL HOSPITAL BOARD, SCOTLAND (1967). *Nursing Workload as a Basis for Staffing.* Scottish health Service Studies No. 3. Edinburgh: Scottish Home and health Department.

30. WORK STUDY DEPARTMENT, NORTH EASTERN REGIONAL HOSPITAL BOARD, SCOTLAND (1969). *Nursing Workload per Patient as a Basis for Staffing.* Scottish Health Service Studies No. 9. Edinburgh: Scottish Home and Health Department.

31. WORK STUDY DEPARTMENT, NORTH EASTERN REGIONAL HOSPITAL BOARD, SCOTLAND (1967). *Nursing Workload as a Basis for Staffing.* Scottish Health Service Studies No. 9, p. 1. Edinburgh: Scottish Home and Health Department.

32. WORK STUDY DEPARTMENT, NORTH EASTERN REGIONAL HOSPITAL BOARD, SCOTLAND (1969). *Nursing Workload per Patient as a Basis for Staffing.* Scottish Health Service Studies No. 9, p. 24. Edinburgh: Scottish Home and Health Department.

33. BRYANT Y. M. and HERON, K. (1974). Monitoring Patient—Nurse Dependency. *Nursing Times.* Vol. 70, pp. 1–7. (Occasional Papers.)

34. IBID., p. 2.

35. IBID., p. 7.

36. IBID.

37. HEARN, C. R. (1974). Evaluation of Patients' Nursing Needs: Prediction of Staffing 1, 2, 3, 4. *Nursing Times.* Vol. 70, p. 1. (Occasional Papers.)

38. IBID., p. 2.

39. IBID., p. 5.
40. IBID., pp. 6–7.
41. IBID., p. 7.
42. OPERATIONAL RESEARCH UNIT, OXFORD REGIONAL HOSPITAL BOARD (1967). *Measurement of Nursing Care,* No. 9. Oxford: Oxford Regional Hospital Board.
43. WORK STUDY DEPARTMENT, NORTH EASTERN REGIONAL HOSPITAL BOARD, SCOTLAND (1967). *Nursing Workload as Basis for Staffing.* Scottish Health Service Studies, No. 3. Edinburgh: Scottish Home and Health department.
44. WORK STUDY DEPARTMENT, NORTH EASTERN REGIONAL HOSPITAL BOARD, SCOTLAND (1969). *Nursing Workload per Patient as a Basis for Staffing.* Scottish Health Service Studies, No. 9. Edinburgh: Scottish Home and Health Department.
45. EASTERN REGIONAL HOSPITAL BOARD (1973). *Instruction Manual. Patient Dependency.* Dundee: Eastern Regional Hospital Board.
46. AULD, M. (1974). *A Method of Estimating the Requisite Nursing Establishment.* M. Phil. Thesis, University of Edinburgh. (Unpublished.)
47. FREDERICK, J. and NORTHAN, E. (1938). *A Texboook of Nursing Practice,* p. 41. New York: MacMillan Co.
48. KING, E. M. (1968). A Conceptual Frame of Reference for Nursing. *Nursing Research.* Vol 17, No. 1, pp. 27–31.
49. HENDERSON, V. (1969). *ICN Basic Principles of Nursing Care.* p. 4. Basel: S. Krager.
50. IBID.
51. IBID., p. 12.
52. NEMO (1973). Tender Loving Care. *Nursing Times,* Vol. 69, No. 27, p. 876.
53. EATON, S. (1966). Have We Lost Our Vision? *Nursing Times,* Vol. 62, No. 36, p. 1167.
54. DOLAN, V. (1973). The Real Case for T.L.C. *Nursing Times,* Vol. 69, No. 40, p. 306.
55. SINTON, J. (1974). Were You There? The Old Man. *Nursing Mirror,* Vol. 138, No. 3, p. 72.
56. HARTSHORN, M. (1974). Don't Talk Over Their Heads. *Nursing Times,* Vol. 70, No. 16, pp. 605–7.
57. JELL, F. E. (1975). I Went Into Hospital. *Nursing Mirror,* Vol. 140, No. 14, p. 67.
58. GOODWIN, P. (1975). The Need for Compassion. *Nursing Mirror,* Vol. 141, No. 24, p. 11.
59. BENDALL, E. R. D. (1973). Education for Change. *Nursing Mirror,* Vol. 137, No. 11, p. 39.
60. SCHMACH, J. A. (1964). Ritualism in Nursing Practice. *Nursing Forum,* Vol. III, No. 4, p. 74.
61. BOYLAN, A. (1974). An Approach to Nursing—1. Developing Clinical Expertise. *Nursing Times,* Vol. 70, No. 46, pp. 1780–1.
62. LELEAN, S. (1973). *Ready for Report Nurse?* The Study of Nursing Care, Series 2, No. 2, p. 116. London: Royal College of Nursing of the United Kingdom.
63. PEMBREY, S. (1975). From Work Routines to Patient Assignment, an Experiment in Ward Administration. *Nursing Times,* Vol. 71, No. 45, pp. 1768–72.

64. HEALY, K. M. (1968). Does a Preoperative Instruction make a Difference? *American Journal of Nursing.* Vol. 68, pp. 62–7.
65. HAYWARD, J. (1975). *Information—A Prescription Against Pain.* A Study of Nursing Care, Series 2, Number 5, London: Royal College of Nursing of the United Kingdom.
66. DUMAS, R. G. and LEONARD, R. C. (1963). Effect of Nursing on the Incidence of Post-Operative Vomiting—A Clinical Experiment. *Nursing Research,* Vol. 12, pp. 12–15.
67. ELMS, R. R. and LEONARD, R. C. (1966). Effects of Nursing Approaches During Admission. *Nursing Research,* Vol. 15, No. 1, pp. 39–47.
68. WOLFER, J. A. and VISINTAINER, M. A. (1975). Pediatric Surgical Patients' and Parents' Stress Responses and Adjustment as a Function of Psychological Preparation and Stress—Point Nursing Care. *Nursing Research,* Vol. 24, No. 4, pp. 244–55.
69. TIERNEY, A. (1973). Toilet Training. *Nursing Times,* Vol. 20, No. 27, pp. 1740–5.
70. IBID., p. 1743.
71. IBID., p. 1743.
72. HOLDER, S. (1973). Rediscovering the Patient. *Nursing Times,* Vol. 69, No. 40, p. 1275.
73. CIUCA, R. L. (1972). Over the Years with the Nursing Care Plan. *Nursing Outlook,* Vol. 20, No. 11, pp. 706–11.
74. IBID., p. 706.
75. IBID., p. 706.
76. IBID., p. 708.
77. MORGAN, D. M. (1974). A Check System for Nursing Care, *Dimensions in Health Service,* Vol. 51, pp. 10–12.
78. CIUCA, R. L. (1972). Over the Years with the Nursing Care Plan. *Nursing Outlook,* Vol. 20, No. 11, p. 706.
79. MANSFIELD, E. (1968). Care Plans to Stimulate Learning. *American Journal of Nursing,* Vol. 68, No. 12, pp. 2592–3.
80. HENDERSON, V. (1969). *I.C.N. Basic Principles of Nursing Care,* p. 4, Basel: S. Krager.
81. WAGNER, B. (1961). The Nursing Care Plan. *Nursing Outlook,* Vol. 9, No. 3, p. 172.
82. SWEET, P. R. and STARK, I. (1970). The Circular Nursing Care Plan. *American Journal of Nursing,* Vol. 70, No. 6, p. 1300.
83. SWEET, P. R. and Stark, I. (1970). The Circular Nursing Care Plan. *American Journal of Nursing,* Vol. 70, No. 6, p. 1300.
84. KING'S FUND CENTRE (1974). *Nurses Reporting on Patients.* Report of a Meeting held at the King's Fund Centre, 4 February, 1974. London: K.F.C. Report No. 858.
85. CIUCA, R. L. (1972). Over the Years with the Nursing Care Plan. *Nursing Outlook,* Vol. 20, No. 11, p. 706.
86. WAGNER, B. (1961). The Nursing Care Plan. *Nursing Outlook,* Vol. 9, No. 3, p. 172.
87. KELLY, N. C. (1966). Nursing Care Plans. *Nursing Outlook,* Vol. 14, No. 5, p. 61.
88. COPP, L. A. (1972). Improved Patient Care Through Evaluation, Part 3. Your Plan of Nursing Care. *Bedside Nurse,* September, 1972, p. 12.

89. WAGNER, B. (1969). Care Plans, Right, Reasonable and Reachable. *American Journal of Nursing*, Vol. 69, No. 5, pp. 986–90.
90. PALISIN, H. (1971). Nursing Care Plans are a Snare and a Delusion. *American Journal of Nursing*, Vol. 71, No. 1, p. 63.
91. NURSING CARE PLAN COMMITTEE (1973). Minutes of Meeting held at North Lothian Region on March 21 and 22, 1973. (Unpublished.)
92. INTERNATIONAL LABOUR OFFICE (1968). *Introduction to Work Study*, p. 262. Geneva: International Labour Office.
93. IBID., p. 247.
94. IBID., p. 261.
95. LEEDS REGIONAL HOSPITAL BOARD (1963). *Work Measurement as a Basis for Calculating Nursing Establishments*, p. 8, Leeds: Leeds Regional Hospital Board.

Bibliography—Books

ABDELLAH, F., BELAND, I. L., Martin, A. and MALHENEY, R. (1960). *Patient-Centred Approaches to Nursing.* New York: The MacMillan Co.

ABEL, P., FARMER, P. J., HUNTER, M. H. S. and SHIPP, P. J. (1974). *National Nursing Manpower Policies in Scotland.* Edinburgh: Institute for Operational Research. Tavistock Institute of Human Relations.

AULD, M. (1974). *A Method of Estimating the Requisite Nursing Establishment.* M. Phil. Thesis, University of Edinburgh. (Unpublished.)

AYDELOTTE, M. K. (1973). *Nurse Staff Methodology. A Review and Critique of Selected Literature.* Washington, D.C.: U.S. Department of Health, Education and Welfare.

BANKS, I. (1972). *Nurse Allocation.* London: William Heinemann, Medical Books Ltd.

DEPARTMENT OF HEALTH AND SOCIAL SECURITY, SCOTTISH HOME AND HEALTH DEPARTMENT AND WELSH OFFICE (1972). *Report of the Committee on Nursing.* London: HMSO. Cmnd. 5115.

DIVISION OF NURSING, DEPARTMENT OF HEALTH, EDUCATION AND WELFARE (1972). *Planning for Nursing Needs and Resources.* DHEW Public. No. (NIH) 72–87, April, 1972. U.S. Department of Health, Education and Welfare. Division of Nursing Selected Publications.

EXTON-SMITH, A. N., NORTON, D. and McLAREN, R. (1962). *Investigation of Geriatric Nursing Problems in Hospital, Part II. Pressure Sores.* London: National Corporation for the Care of Old People.

FREDERICK, H. and NORTHAM, E. (1938). *A Textbook of Nursing Practice.* New York: The MacMillan Co.

HAYWARD, J. (1975). *Information—A Prescription Against Pain. A Study of Nursing Care.* Series 2. Number 5. London: Royal College of Nursing of the United Kingdom.

HENDERSON, V. (1969). *I.C.N. Basic Principles of Nursing Care.* Basel: S. Krager.

INTERNATIONAL LABOUR OFFICE (1968). *Introduction to Work Study,* Geneva: International Labour Office.

JEFFERY, I. J. and LOWE, S. M. (1963). *Patient-Nurse Dependency Exploratory Study.* SP. Report 11. Operational Research Unit, Wellington: Department of Health. N.2.

KING EDWARD'S HOSPITAL FUND FOR LONDON (1945). *Considerations of Standards of Staffing.* Cited by: The Nuffield Provincial Hospitals Trust (1953). *The Work of Nurses in Hospital Wards.* London: The Nuffield Provincial Hospitals Trust.

KRON, T. (1961). *Nursing Team Leadership.* Philadelphia: W.B. Saunders Co.

LAMBERTSON, E. C. (1958). *Education for Nursing Leadership.* Philadelphia: J.B. Lippincott.

LARKIN, J. A. (1969). *Work Study. Theory and Practice.* London: McGraw-Hill.

178

LEEDS REGIONAL HOSPITAL BOARD (1963). *Work Measurement as a Basis for Calculating Nursing Establishments*. Leeds: Regional Hospital Board.

LELEAN, S. (1973). *Ready for Report Nurse?* The Study of Nursing Care. Series 2. No. 2. London: Royal College of Nursing of the United Kingdom.

LEVINE, E. (ed.) (1972). *Research on Nurse Staffing in Hospitals*. Report of the Conference conducted by the Division of Nursing. DHEW Publication, No. (NH.) 73–434. Washington, D.C.: U.S. Department of Health, Education and Welfare. Public Health Service. National Institutes of Health, Bureau of Health Manpower. Division of Nursing.

LUCK, G. M., et al. (1971). *Patients Hospitals and Operational Research*. London: Tavistock Publications.

MCFARLANE, J. K. (1970). *The Proper Study of the Nurse*. London: Royal College of Nursing.

MCLACHLAN, G. (ed.) (1964). *Problems and Progress in Medical Care: Essays on Current Research*. London: Published for the Nuffield Provincial Hospitals Trust by the Oxford University Press.

MCLACHLAN, G. (ed.) (1973). *The Future and Present Indicatives*. Problems and Progress in Medical Care Series 9. London: Oxford University Press for the Nuffield Provincial Hospitals Trust.

MCLACHLAN, G. and SEGOG, R. A. (1968). *Computer in the Service of Medicine*. I and II. London: Oxford University Press for the Nuffield provincial Hospitals Trust.

MARRAM, G. D., SCHLEGEL, M. and BEVIS, E. O. (1974). *Primary Nursing: A Model for Individualised Care*. Saint Louis: The C. V. Mosby Co.

THE NUFFIELD PROVINCIAL HOSPITALS TRUST (1953). *The Work of Nurses in Hospital Wards. Report of a Job-Analysis*. London: The Nuffield Provincial Hospitals Trust.

NUFFIELD PROVINCIAL HOSPITALS TRUST (1973). *The Future and Present Indicatives. Problems and Progress in Medical Care. Essays on Current Research*. London: Oxford University Press.

NURSING UNIT, WORLD HEALTH ORGANISATION (1970). *Nursing Manpower Development—A Review of Methods*. Prepared for the Scientific Group on the Development of Studies in Health Manpower held in Geneva, 2–10 November, 1970. W.H.O./Nurs/71.79.

OCKENDEN, J. M. and BODENHAM, K. E. (1970). *Focus on Medical Computer Development*. London: Nuffield Provincial Hospitals Trust and Oxford University Press.

OPERATIONAL RESEARCH UNIT, OXFORD REGIONAL HOSPITAL BOARD (1967). *Measurement of Nursing Care*. No. 9. Oxford Regional Hospital Board.

OPERATIONAL RESEARCH UNIT, OXFORD REGIONAL HOSPITAL BOARD (1970). *Nursing Care in a Modern Hospital*. Oxford: Oxford Regional Hospital Board.

PAETZNICK, M. (1966). *A Guide for Staffing a Hospital Nursing Service*. Geneva: World Health Organisation.

PAYNE, L. C. (1966). *An Introduction to Medical Automation*. London: Pitman Medical.

WHITBY, L. G. and LUTZ, W. (eds.) (1971). *Principles and Practice of Medical Computing*. Edinburgh: Churchill Livingstone.

WORK STUDY DEPARTMENT, NORTH EASTERN REGIONAL HOSPITAL BOARD, SCOTLAND (1967). *Nursing Workload as a Basis for Staffing*. Scottish

Health Services Studies No. 3. Edinburgh: Scottish Home and Health Department.

WORK STUDY DEPARTMENT, NORTH EASTERN REGIONAL HOSPITAL BOARD, SCOTLAND (1969). *Nursing Workload per Patient as a Basis for Staffing.* Scottish Health Service Series No. 9. Edinburgh: Scottish Home and Health Department.

Bibliography—Periodicals

AIKEN, L. H. and HENRICHS, T. F. (1971). Systematic Relaxation on a Nursing Intervention Technique with Open Heart Surgery Patients. *Nursing Research.* Vol. 20, No. 3, p. 212.

BALDWIN, S. M. (1976). Made to Measure Care. *Nursing Times.* Vol. 72, No. 12, pp. 468–9.

BARLOW, A. J. (1972). Nurse Allocation by Computer. *Nursing Mirror.* Vol. 134, No. 4, pp. 43–5.

BARNETT, D. (1975). Standards of Nursing Care—Why are They Falling? *Nursing Mirror.* Vol. 140, No. 24, pp. 58–60.

BARR, A. et al. (1973). A Review of the Various Methods of Measuring the Dependency of Patients on Nursing Staff. *International Journal of Nursing Studies.* Vol. 10, No. 3, pp. 195–208.

BEAT, J. W. S. (1970). Ward Analysis. *Nursing Times,* Vol. 66, No. 29, p. 101.

BENDALL, E. R. D. (1973). Education for Change. *Nursing Mirror.* Vol. 137, No. 11, p. 39.

BOORE, J. (1975). The Planning of Nursing Care. *Nursing Mirror.* Vol. 141, No. 15, pp. 59–61.

BOYLAN, A. (1974). An Approach to Nursing—1. Developing Clinical Expertise. *Nursing Times.* Vol. 70, No. 46, p. 1780.

BRINHAM, R. O. J. (1972). Looking at Ward Activity. *Nursing Times.* Vol. 68, No. 37, pp. 1154–5.

BROWN, P. T. (1970). Computers and the Nurse. *International Journal of Nursing Studies.* Vol. 7, No. 2, p. 91.

BROWN, R. L. (1976). Cumputerised Nursing. *Nursing Mirror.* Vol. 142, No. 6, p. 56.

BRYANT, Y. M. and HERON, K. (1974). Monitoring Patient-Nurse Dependency. *Nursing Times.* Vol. 70, pp. 1–7. (Occasional Papers).

BURCH, M. (1975). Teaching in the Ward Environment. *Nursing Mirror.* Vol. 141, No. 5, pp. 59–61.

BUTLER, E. A. (1973). Computers in the Ward Situation. *Nursing Times.* Vol. 69, No. 4, pp. 119–21.

CIUCA, R. L. (1972). Over the Years with the Nursing Care Plans. *Nursing Outlook.* Vol. 20, No. 11, p. 706.

COLLEDGE, M. (1973). Cooling the Mark Out a Nursing Function. *Nursing Times.* Vol. 69, No. 36, pp. 1157–8.

COPP, L. A. (1972). Improved Patient Care Through Evaluation. Part 3. Your Plan of Nursing Care. *Bedside Nurse.* September, 1972, p. 12.

CORNELL, S. A. and BRUSH, F. (1971). Systems Approach to Nursing Care Plans. *American Journal of Nursing.* Vol. 71, No. 7, pp. 1376–8.

CORNELL, S. A. and CARRICK, A. G. (1973). Computerised Schedules and Care Plans. *Nursing Outlook.* Vol. 12, No. 12, pp. 781–4.

COWPER-SMITH, F. (1976). The Intangible Line. *Nursing Times.* Vol. 72, No. 51, p. 2021.

CROOKS, J. (1976). Drug administration—2. *Nursing Mirror,* Vol. 142, No. 14, pp. 55–7.

CROOKS, J. and HEDLEY, T. (1974). The Information Deep Freeze. *Computing Europe.* August 22, 1974, pp. 11–13.

CROSSLEY, J. R. (1974). Nursing and Midwifery Resources and Their Utilisation. *Nightingale Fellowship Journal.* Vol. 90, pp. 518–24.

DANIELS, S. (1972). What Are Nursing Duties? *Nursing Times,* Vol. 68, No. 4, p. 121.

DAVID, M. and SAUNDERS, R. (1966). Allocating Student Nurses by Computer. *Nursing Times.* Vol. 62, No. 14, p. 467

DOLAN, V. (1973). The Real Case for T.L.C. *Nursing Times.* Vol. 69, No. 50, p. 306.

DUMAS, R. G. and LEONARD R. C. (1963). Effect of Nursing on the Incidence of Post-Operative Vomiting—A Clinical Experiment. *Nursing Research.* Vol. 12, p. 12.

EATON, S. (1966). Have We Lost Our Vision? *Nursing Times.* Vol. 62, No. 36, p. 1167.

EDITORIAL. (1973). An Ostrich Attitude. *Nursing Times.* Vol. 69, No. 36, p. 1139.

ELMS, R. R. and LEONARD, R. C. (1966) Effects of Nursing Approaches During Admission. *Nursing Research.* Vol. 15, No. 1, p. 39.

FARLEE, C. and GOLDSTEIN, B. (1971). A Role for Nurses in Implementing Computerised Hospital Information Systems. *Nursing Forum.* Vol. X, No. 4, p. 339.

FULD, M. (1066). Swollen Legs, Causes Diagnosed by Computer and Conventionally. *Nursing Times.* Vol. 62, No. 15, pp. 511–3.

FEYERHERM, A. M. (1966). Nursing Activity Patterns: A Guide to Staffing. *Nursing Research.* Vol. 15, No. 2, pp. 124–33.

FINE, R. B. (1974). Controlling Nurses' Workloads. *American Journal of Nursing.* Vol. 74, No. 12, pp. 2206–7.

FLINT, R. T. and SPENSLEY, K. C. (1969). Recent Issues in Nursing Manpower: A Review. *Nursing Pesearch.* Vol. 18, No. 3, pp. 217–29.

FOSTER, V. L. (1961). The Night Nurse is Very Special. *Nursing Outlook.* Vol. 9, No. 12, pp. 765–6.

GARANT, C. (1972). A Basic for Care. *American Journal of Nursing.* Vol. 72, pp. 699–701.

GOODWIN, J. O. and EDWARDS, B. S. (1975). Developing a Computer Programme to Assist the Nursing Process: Phase I—From Systems Analysis to an Expandable Programme. *Nursing Research.* Vol. 24, No. 4, pp. 299–305.

GOODWIN, P. (1975). The Need for Compassion. *Nursing Mirror.* Vol. 141, No. 24, p. 11.

GRAZMAN, T. E. (1969). Manpower Utilisation Study Reflects Personnel Requirements. *Hospitals.* Vol. 43, pp. 82–6.

GRIFFITH, R. (1974). Nursing in the Home—A Suitable Case for Treatment. *Computing Europe.* October 10, 1974.

H. S. HALEUI, and RON, R. (1976). Medical Patient/Nurse Dependency in Israel. *Journal of Advanced Nursing.* Vol. 1, No. 1, pp. 63/78.

HALL, L. E. (1969). The LOEB Center for Nursing and Rehabilitation, Montefiore Hospital and Medical Center, Bronx, New York. *International Journal of Nursing Studies.* Vol. 6, pp. 81–97.

HANNAH, K. J. (1976) The Computer and Nursing Practice. *Nursing Outlook.* Vol. 24, No. 9, pp. 555–8.

HARDIE, M. W. (1975). Geriatrics Patient Care. *Nursing Times.* Vol. 71, pp. 61–4. (Occasional Papers).

HARGREAVES, I. (1975). The Nursing Process. The Key to Individualised Care. *Nursing Times.* Vol. 71, No. 35, pp. 89–92.

HARRIS, B. L. (1970). Who Needs Written Care Plans Anyway? *American Journal of Nursing.* Vol. 70, No. 10, pp. 21–37.

HARTMANN, B. (1968). Student Nurse Allocation. *Nursing Times.* Vol. 64, pp. 1–4. (Occasional Papers).

HARTSHORNE, M. (1974). Don't Talk Over Their Heads. *Nursing Times.* Vol. 70, No. 16, p. 605.

HASSELL, D. (1971). Patient Dependency Related to Nurse Staffing In A.M.S. Hospital: 1 and 2. *Nursing Times.* Vol. 67, pp. 77–84. (Occasional Papers).

HAUSSMAN, R. K. et al. (1974). Monitering Quality of Nursing Care. *Health Services Research.* Summer 1974. Vol. 9, No. 2, pp. 135–47.

HEAD, A. E. (1977). Keeping the Ward Records Straight. *Computer Weekly.* February 3, 1977.

HEALY, K. M. (1968). Does a Preoperative Instruction Make a Difference. *American Journal of Nursing.* Vol. 68, p. 62.

HENDERSON, V. (1973). Nursing Care Plans and Their History. *Nursing Outlook.* Vol. 21, pp. 378–9.

HENNEY, C. (1975). Drug Administration—1. *Nursing Mirror.* Vol. 142, No. 14, pp. 52–4.

HUMPHRIES, J. (1975). A Life Worth Living. *Nursing Times,* Vol. 71, No. 42, pp. 1661–2.

HOLDER, S. (1973). Rediscovering the Patient. *Nursing Times.* Vol. 69, No. 40, p. 1275.

JELL, F. E. (1975). I Went Into Hospital. *Nursing Mirror,* Vol. 140, No. 14, p. 67.

KAHOSHI, M. E. (1957). A Method of Studying the Utilisation of Nursing Service Personnel in Veterans Administration Hospital. *Nursing Research.* Vol. 61, No. 2, pp. 79–81.

KELLY, N. C. (1966). Nursing Care Plans. *Nursing Outlook.* Vol. 14, No. 5, p. 61.

KENNEDY, F. (1970). Switch—Hospital Case History on Computer. *Scottish Medical Journal.* Vol. 15, pp. 391–4.

KING, I. M. (1968). A Conceptual Frame of Reference for Nursing. *Nursing Research.* Vol. 17, No. 1, pp. 27–31.

KING'S FUND CENTRE (1974). *Nursing Reporting on Patients.* Report of a Meeting Held at the King's Fund Centre, 4 February, 1974, K.F.C. Report No. 858.

KNIGHT, J. E. and STREETER, J. (1970). The Computer as an Aid to Nursing Records. *Nursing Times.* Vol. 66, No. 8, p. 233.

KEAEGEL, J. M. et al. (1972). A System of Patient Care Based on Patient Needs. *Nursing Outlook.* Vol. 20, No. 4, pp. 257–64.

LAGINA, S. M. (1971). A Computer to Diagnose Anxiety Levels. *Nursing Research.* Vol. 20, No. 6, p. 484.

LINDEMAN, C. A. and VAN AERNAM, B.(1971). Nursing Intervention with the Pre-Surgical Patient—the Effects of Structured and Unstructured Pre-Operative Teaching. *Nursing Research.* Vol. 20, No. 4, pp. 320–2.

183

LITTLE, D. and CARNEVALI, D. (1971). The Nursing Care Planning System. *Nursing Outlook*. Vol. 19, pp. 164–7.

McFARLANE, J. K. (1975). What Do We Mean By Care. *Nursing Mirror*. Vol. 141, No. 14, pp. 47–8.

McFARLANE, J. K. (1975). A Charter for Caring. *Nursing Mirror*. Vol. 141, No. 23, pp. 40–2.

MAGUIRE, G. P. et. al. (1974). Psychiatric Morbidity and Referral on Two General Medical Wards. *The British Medical Journal*. 1974. No. 1; 268–70.

MANSFIELD, E. (1968). Care Plans to Stimulate Learning. *American Journal of Nursing*. Vol. 68, No. 12, p. 2592.

MATTHEWS, A. (1975). Patient Allocation. A Review. *Nursing Times*. Vol. 71, No. 28, pp. 65–8.

MEATES, D. (1972). The Diminishing Island of Nursing Duties. *Nursing Times*. Vol. 68, no. 43, p. 1348.

MILLER, E. A. (1976). Staffing with the Aid of Dependency Indices. *Nursing Times*. Vol. 72, No. 32, pp. 113–115. (Occasional Paper).

MITCHELL, J. H. (1969). Relevance of the Electronic Computer to Hospital Medical Records. *British Medical Journal*. 1969. No. 4, pp. 157–9

MOORE, P. and CARR, J. (1976). Behaviour Modification Programme. *Nursing Times*. Vol. 72, No. 35, pp. 1356–9.

MORGAN, D. M. (1974). A Check System for Nursing Care. *Dimensions in Health Service*. Vol. 51, p. 10.

MULLIGAN, B. (1972). How Many Nurses Equal Enough? *Nursing Times*. Vol. 68, No. 15, pp. 428–30.

MURPHY, J. (1975). The Role of the Ward Sister. *Nursing Mirror*. Vol. 140, No. 7, pp. 71–2.

NEMO (1973). Tender Loving Care. *Nursing Times,* Vol. 69, No. 27, p. 876.

NORWICH, H. S. and SENIOR, O. E. (1971). Determining Nursing Establishment. *Nursing Times*. Vol. 67, No. 5, pp. 17–20. (Occasional Papers).

NURSING MIRROR. (1973). Computer Check on Drug Reactions. *Nursing Mirror*. Vol. 136, No. 12, pp. 31.

NURSING TIMES. (1973). Radical Plan to Cope with Nursing Shortage. *Nursing Times*. Vol. 69, No. 50, p. 1673.

NURSING MIRROR. (1975). Probe to Match Nurses with Needs. *Nursing Mirror*. Vol. 141, No. 22, p. 35.

NURSING TIMES. (1975). Fully Understaffed. *Nursing Times*. Vol. 71, No. 42, p. 1637.

OPIT, L. J. and WOODROOFE, F. J. (1970). Computer-Held Clinical Record System. *British Medical Journal*. 1970, No. 4, pp. 76–82.

OSBORNE, M. (1970). Computer in Psychiatry. *Canadian Nurse*. Vol. 66, No. 10, pp. 39–40.

PALISIN, H. (1971). Nursing Care Plans are a Snare and a Delusion. *American Journal of Nursing*. Vol. 71, No. 1, p. 63.

PARDEE, G. et. al. (1971). Patient Care Evaluation is Every Nurse's Job. *American Journal of Nursing*. Vol. 71, pp. 1958–60.

PAYNE, L. C. (1965). Computers and Patient Management. *Nursing Times*. Vol. 61, No. 39, pp. 1339–41.

PAYNE, L. C. (1965). Medical Automation, A. Proffesional Necessity. *Nursing Mirror*. Vol. 120, No. 3123, p.v.

PEMBREY, S. 1975). From Work Routines to Patient Assignment, An Experiment in Ward Administration. *Nursing Times*. Vol. 71, No. 45, p. 1768.

PEPLAU, H. E. (1960). Talking with Patients. *American Journal of Nursing*. Vol. 60, No. 7, pp. 964–6.

PHILLIPS, D. (1975). The Patient is Person. *Nursing Mirror*. Vol. 141, No. 4, pp. 64–5.

PRICE, J. (1972). Patient Care Classification System. *Nursing Outlook*. Vol. 20, No. 7, pp. 445–8.

RHYS-HEARN C. (1974). Evaluation of Patients' Nursing Needs: Prediction of Staffing 1, 2, 3, 4. *Nursing Times*. Vol. 70. pp. 69–84. (Occasional Papers).

RHYS-HEARN, C. (1972). Evaluating Patients' Nursing Needs. *Nursing Times*. Vol. 68, pp. 65–68.

RHYS-HEARN, C. (1972). How Many High Care Patients. How Birmingham Tackles the Problem—1, 2. *Nursing Times*. Vol. 68, No. 16, pp. 472–4. No. 17, pp. 504–5.

RUDD, T. N. (1974). Improving the Quality of Life in Hospital. *Nursing Mirror*. Vol. 139, No. 23, pp. 53–4.

RUSHWORTH, V. (1975). Manpower Planning at District Level. *Nursing Times*. Vol. 71, No. 51, pp. 2032–3.

SAFFORD, B. J. and SCHLOFELDT, R. M. (1960). Nursing Service Staffing and Quality of Nursing Care. *Nursing Research*. Vol. 9, pp. 149–54.

SCHMACH, J. A. (1964). Ritualism in Nursing Practice. *Nursing Forum*. Vol. III, No. 4, p. 74.

SCHOLES, M. (1976). The Role of Computers in Nursing. *Nursing Mirror*. Vol. 143, No. 13, pp. 46–8.

SKEET, M. (1974). Talking to Patients. *Nursing Mirror*. Vol. 138, No. 7, p. 44.

SMITH, B. (1970). Computer in the Ward. *Nursing Times*. Vol. 66, No. 45, p. 1426.

SINTON, J. (1974). Were You There? The Old Man. *Nursing Mirror*. Vol. 138, No. 3, p. 72.

SOMERS, J. B. (1971). A Computerised Nursing Care System. *Hospitals*. Vol. 45, pp. 93–100.

SPEED, E. L. and YOUNG, N. A. (1969). Scan Data Processed Printouts of a Patient's Basic Care Needs. *American Journals of Nursing*. Vol. 69, No. 1, pp. 108–10.

STUBBER, B. F. (1975). Team Nursing—Why? *Nursing Mirror*. Vol. 141, No. 11, p. 72.

STURLIE, F. (1970). Nursing Need Never Be Defined. *International Nursing Review*. Vol. 17, No. 3, pp. 254–7.

SWEET, P. R. and STARK, I. (1970). The Circular Nursing Care Plan. *American Journal of Nursing*. Vol. 70, No. 6, p. 1300.

THE SCOTSMAN. (1973). Nursing: A Suitable Case for Treatment. *The Scotsman*. November 6, 1973.

THORNTON, M. (1975). The Giving of Care. *Nursing Mirror*. Vol. 141, No. 15, pp. 62–3.

TIERNEY, A. (1973). Toilet Training. *Nursing Times*. Vol. 20, No. 27, p. 1740.

TINKER, J. (1973). Information for Intensive Care. *Nursing Mirror*. Vol. 136, No. 14, p. 34.

TRIVEDI, V. M. and HANCOCK, W. M. (1975). Measurement of Nursing Workload Using Head Nurses Perceptions. *Nursing Research.* Vol. 24, No. 5, pp. 371–6.

WAGNER, B. (1961). The Nursing Care Plan. *Nursing Outlook.* Vol. 9, No. 3, p. 172.

WAGNER, B. (1969). Care Plans, Right, Reasonable and Reachable. *American Journal of Nursing.* Vol. 69, No. 5, p. 986.

WALSH, M. (1975). R.C.N. Student Nurses Share Concern for Quality of Patient Care. *Nursing Mirror.* Vol. 141, No. 13, p. 35.

WASKETT, C. (1973). Nursing Mr. James. *Nursing Times.* Vol. 69, No. 48, p. 1640.

WESSELING, E. (1972). Automating the Nursing History and Care Plan. *Journal of Nursing Administration.* Vol. 2, pp. 34–8. (May-June, 1972).

WILLIAMS, D. (1969). The Administrative Contribution of the Nursing Sister. *Public Administration,* Autumn, 1969, pp. 301–2.

WOLFE, H. and YOUNG, J. P. (1963). Staffing the Nursing Unit: Part One: Controlled Variable Staffing. *Nursing Research,* Vol. 14, p. 237.

WOLFER, J. A. and DAVIS, G. E. (1970). Assessment of Surgical Patients' Preoperative Emotional Condition and Post Operative Welfare. *Nursing Research.* Vol. 19, No. 5, p. 402.

WOLFER, J. A. and VINISTAINER, M. A. (1975). Pediatric Surgical Patients' and Parents' Stress Responses and Adjustment as a Function of Psychological Preparation and Stress—Point Nursing Care. *Nursing Research,* Vol. 24, No. 4, p. 244.